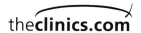

theclinics.com

CLINICS IN LABORATORY MEDICINE

Pharmacogenetics

GUEST EDITORS
Kristen K. Reynolds, PhD
Roland Valdes, Jr, PhD, FACB

CONSULTING EDITOR
Alan Wells, MD, DMSc

December 2008 • Volume 28 • Number 4

SAUNDERS

An Imprint of Elsevier, Inc.
PHILADELPHIA   LONDON   TORONTO   MONTREAL   SYDNEY   TOKYO

W.B. SAUNDERS COMPANY
A Division of Elsevier Inc.

Elsevier, Inc. • 1600 John F. Kennedy Blvd., Suite 1800 • Philadelphia, Pennsylvania 19103-2899

http://www.theclinics.com

CLINICS IN LABORATORY MEDICINE
December 2008
Editor: Joanne Husovski
Developmental Editor: Donald Mumford

Volume 28, Number 4
ISSN 0272-2712
ISBN-13: 978-1-4160-6313-1
ISBN-10: 1-4160-6313-7

Reprints: For copies of 100 or more, of articles in this publication, please contact the Commercial Reprints Department, Elsevier Inc., 360 Park Avenue South, New York, New York 10010-1710. Tel. (212) 633-3813, Fax: (212) 462-1935, e-mail: reprints@elsevier.com.

Clinics in Laboratory Medicine (ISSN 0272-2712) is published quarterly by Elsevier Inc., 360 Park Avenue South, New York, NY 10010-1710. Months of issue are March, June, September, and December. Business and Editorial offices: 1600 John F. Kennedy Blvd., Suite 1800, Philadelphia, PA 19103-2899. Customer Service Office: 6277 Sea Harbor Drive, Orlando, FL 32887-4800. Periodicals postage paid at New York, NY and additional mailing offices. Subscription prices are $204.00 per year (US individuals), $321.00 per year (US institutions), $106.00 (US students), $234.00 per year (Canadian individuals), $405.00 per year (foreign institutions), $145.00 (foreign students). Foreign air speed delivery is included in all *Clinics* subscription prices. All prices are subject to change without notice. POSTMASTER: Send address changes to *Clinics in Laboratory Medicine*, Elsevier Periodicals Customer Service 11830 Westline Industrial Drive St. Louis, MO 63146. **Customer Service: 1-800-654-2452 (US). From outside of the US, call 1-314-453-7041. Fax: 1-314-453-5170. E-mail: JournalsCustomerService-usa@elsevier.com (for print support) or journalsonlinesupport-usa@elsevier.com (for online support).**

Clinics in Laboratory Medicine is covered in *EMBASE/Exerpta Medica, MEDLINE/PubMed (Index Medicus), Cinahl, Current Contents/Clinical Medicine, BIOSIS* and *ISI/BIOMED.*

Printed in the United States of America.

CONSULTING EDITOR

ALAN WELLS, MD, DMSc, Vice Chairman, Department of Pathology, Thomas J. Gill III Professor of Pathology, Medical Director, Section of Laboratory Medicine, University of Pittsburgh, Pittsburgh, Pennsylvania

GUEST EDITORS

KRISTEN K. REYNOLDS, PhD, PG_{XL} Laboratories Vice President, Laboratory Operations; and Assistant Clinical Professor, Department of Pathology and Laboratory Medicine, University of Louisville School of Medicine, Louisville, Kentucky

ROLAND VALDES, Jr, PhD, FACB, Professor and Senior Vice Chairman Department of Pathology and Laboratory Medicine, and Professor of Biochemistry and Molecular Biology, University of Louisville School of Medicine, Louisville, Kentucky

CONTRIBUTORS

ALICIA ALGECIRAS-SCHIMNICH, PhD, Assistant Professor, Division of Clinical Biochemistry and Immunology, Department of Laboratory Medicine and Pathology, College of Medicine, Mayo Clinic, Rochester, Minnesota

MOHAMMAD AL-GHOUL, PhD, Postdoctoral Fellow, Department of Pathology and Laboratory Medicine, University of Louisville School of Medicine, Louisville, Kentucky

MARIA J. ARRANZ, PhD, Senior Lecturer, Clinical Neuropsychopharmacology, Psychological Medicine, Institute of Psychiatry, King's College, London, United Kingdom

MARJORIE BON HOMME, PhD, Department of Pathology and Laboratory Medicine, University of Louisville, Louisville, Kentucky

BONNY LEWIS BUKAVECKAS, PhD, Assistant Professor, Department of Pharmacy; Department of Pathology; and Department of Anesthesiology, School of Pharmacy, Virginia Commonwealth University, Richmond, Virginia

JOSÉ DE LEON, MD, Medical Director, University of Kentucky Mental Health Research Center at Eastern State Hospital; Professor of Psychiatry, University of Kentucky Colleges of Medicine and Pharmacy, Lexington, Kentucky; Visiting Professor and Member of Psychiatry Neurosciences Research Group, Institute of Neurosciences, University of Granada, Granada, Spain

ALEXANDER DUNCAN, MD, Assistant Professor of Pathology and Laboratory Medicine; and Medical Director, Special Coagulation Laboratory, Emory University School of Medicine, Emory University Hospital, Atlanta, Georgia

RIFAAT S. EL-MALLAKH, MD, Professor and Director, Mood Disorders Research Program, Department of Psychiatry and Behavioral Sciences, University of Louisville School of Medicine, Louisville, Kentucky

CHARLES E. HILL, MD, PhD, Assistant Professor of Pathology and Laboratory Medicine; and Director Molecular Diagnostics Laboratory, Emory University School of Medicine, Emory University Hospital, Atlanta, Georgia

SAEED A. JORTANI, PhD, Associate Professor, PG_{XL} Laboratories, Louisville, Kentucky; Department of Pathology and Laboratory Medicine, University of Louisville School of Medicine, Louisville, Kentucky

JULIA KIRCHHEINER, MD, Professor, Institute of Pharmacology of Natural Products and Clinical Pharmacology, University of Ulm, Helmholtzstrasse, Ulm, Germany

MARK W. LINDER, PhD, Department of Pathology and Laboratory Medicine, University of Louisville; and PG_{XL} Laboratories, Louisville, Kentucky

ELAINE LYON, PhD, Associate Professor, Department of Pathology, University of Utah; and ARUP Institute for Clinical and Experimental Pathology, Salt Lake City, Utah

GWEN McMILLIN, PhD, Associate Professor, Department of Pathology, University of Utah; and ARUP Institute for Clinical and Experimental Pathology, Salt Lake City, Utah

ROBERTA MELIS, PhD, Research Scientist, ARUP Institute for Clinical and Experimental Pathology, Salt Lake City, Utah

DENNIS J. O'KANE, PhD, Assistant Professor, Division of Clinical Biochemistry and Immunology, Department of Laboratory Medicine and Pathology, College of Medicine, Mayo Clinic, Rochester, Minnesota

BRONWYN RAMEY-HARTUNG, PhD, Manager of Technology Development, PG_{XL} Laboratories, Louisville, Kentucky

KRISTEN K. REYNOLDS, PhD, PG_{XL} Laboratories Vice President, Laboratory Operations; and Assistant Clinical Professor, Department of Pathology and Laboratory Medicine, University of Louisville School of Medicine, Louisville, Kentucky

GUALBERTO RUAÑO, MD, PhD, CEO, Genomas, Inc., Hartford, Connecticut

ANGELA SEERINGER, MD, Institute of Pharmacology of Natural Products and Clinical Pharmacology, University of Ulm, Helmholtzstrasse, Ulm, Germany

CHRISTINE L.H. SNOZEK, PhD, Assistant Professor, Division of Clinical Biochemistry and Immunology, Department of Laboratory Medicine and Pathology, Mayo Clinic College of Medicine, Rochester Minnesota

ROLAND VALDES, Jr, PhD, FACB, Professor and Senior Vice Chairman Department of Pathology and Laboratory Medicine, and Professor of Biochemistry and Molecular Biology, University of Louisville School of Medicine, Louisville, Kentucky

WENDELL W. WEBER, MD, PhD, Emeritus Professor (Active), Department of Pharmacology, University of Michigan Medical School, Ann Arbor, Michigan

LYNN R. WEBSTER, MD, Medical Director, Lifetree Clinical Research and Pain Clinic, Salt Lake City, Utah

I-WEN YU, MS, Doctoral Student in Pharmacotherapy, Department of Pharmacy, School of Pharmacy, Virginia Commonwealth University, Richmond, Virginia

CONTENTS

This article provides an introduction to the fundamental principles of pharmacokinetics (PK) and pharmacodynamics (PD) as they apply to understanding the application of pharmacogenetics (PGx) in a clinical setting. PGx establishes connections between the disciplines of pharmacology and genetics. As such, one functional component of PGx involves establishing relationships between phenotypes and genotypes with respect to predicting the response of medications in individual patients. The article begins by describing each of the concepts, followed by discussing the clinical utility of PGx and pharmacodynamics in a laboratory medicine setting; it then makes a link with the evolving field of PGx from the perspective of clinical laboratory medicine. Laboratory medicine serves as a catalyst for transitioning PGx into clinical settings, and as such, the article concludes by describing the future role of clinical laboratories in the application of PGx to patient care.

Many of the complexities of human drug response are sufficiently well understood to transform the field of pharmacogenetics from a descriptive science to a predictive science. Clinical application of these markers is currently limited by lack of knowledge about the effects of modifying genes, about their prevalence and risk contribution in different ethnogeographic populations, and by fragmentary information about how genetic factors interact with physiologic or pathologic and other environmental factors. Nevertheless, progress has been notable, as exemplified in the identification of genetic markers predictive of pharmacokinetic variation, and in markers predictive of outcome and therapeutic benefit in the treatment of cancer.

Although used for many years, a detailed understanding of the mechanism of action and metabolism of anticoagulants has become available only recently. After the addition of pharmacogenetic data to the drug label by the U.S. Food and Drug Administration, interest in the pharmacogenetics of warfarin and its clinical application has grown exponentially. Dosing algorithms have been developed and continue to be refined that incorporate the polymorphisms of P450 2C9 and vitamin K epoxide reductase. Widespread adoption of these algorithms has been slow because of factors such as physician education, timely testing, complexity of dosing calculations, dietary variations, and other confounding variables. Although most useful before the first dose, these tests are also being used to explain labile responses to warfarin. Current protocols are capable of predicting a large portion of interindividual dosing variation and, as more data become available, truly personalized dosing of warfarin should be achievable, improving patient safety and clinical efficacy.

With the US Food and Drug Administration's recent label change of warfarin to include genetic testing for warfarin sensitivity, manufacturers are developing assays, and laboratories are offering testing. This article describes the genetic variants for which testing is available. Current technologies and assays are compared, including considerations for laboratories in choosing a method. Finally, laboratory issues that apply to all methods, such as quality control and proficiency testing as well as service issues including turn-around-time requirements are discussed.

This article demonstrates how a dynamic clinical-support tool can guide individualized drug therapy. We use the drug warfarin as a model to demonstrate how pharmacogenetics when combined with fundamental principles of pharmacokinetic and pharmacodynamics can provide a powerful decision-support tool to optimize personalized therapeutics.

likelihood of therapeutic response and their relative risk of experiencing toxicity and other adverse side effects from certain drugs. Such information could arm physicians with the knowledge they need to make appropriate drug and dosing decisions and avoid the lengthy trial-and-error process with which they are faced today. This article describes the current state of pharmacogenetic testing in schizophrenia and posttraumatic stress disorder.

β_2-Agonist medications, such as albuterol and salmeterol, are widely used to treat asthma. However, there are a significant number of poor responders. Poor response may present as decreased lung function, and in extreme cases (a small percentage), patients who have asthma are at increased risk for mortality. A common single nucleotide polymorphism (SNP) in the β_2-adrenergic receptor gene (*ADRB2*) results in an arginine substitution for glycine at amino acid 16 (Arg16→Gly) of the β_2-adrenergic receptor protein. Although this SNP has been associated with increased responsiveness at therapy initiation, it has also been associated with decreased lung function and increased asthma exacerbations with long-term use of β_2-agonists with or without corticosteroids in Caucasians. This pharmacogenetic relationship is less well studied in other ethnic groups. Experts have proposed that regular use of albuterol or salmeterol may be inappropriate for Caucasian asthmatics who have the homozygous *ADRB2* Arg16 genotype.

FORTHCOMING ISSUES

RECENT ISSUES

THE CLINICS ARE NOW AVAILABLE ONLINE!

Access your subscription at:
http://www.theclinics.com

CLINICS IN
LABORATORY
MEDICINE

ELSEVIER
SAUNDERS

Clin Lab Med 28 (2008) xiii–xv

Preface

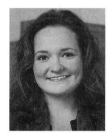 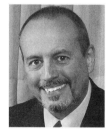

Kristen K. Reynolds, PhD   Roland Valdes, Jr, PhD, FACB
Guest Editors

The series of articles in this issue of *Clinics in Laboratory Medicine* focuses on pharmacogenetics and its application to medicine by way of the clinical laboratory. Research in the area of pharmacogenetics/pharmacogenomics (PGx) has been gaining more attention, as it is now believed to hold part of a solution for several critically important medical problems and is anticipated to form a bridge to personalized medicine in therapeutics. In this series of clinical laboratory medicine reports, several articles discuss aspects of pharmacogenetics in the clinical setting that are related to understanding pharmacogenetics and its application to clinical medicine.

The objective of this issue is to present a basis for understanding the fundamental aspects of pharmacogenetics as related to its applications in anticoagulation, oncology, pain management, and behavioral and respiratory disorders. We begin with an article by Drs. Al-Ghoul and Valdes that provides a framework on which to build an understanding of pharmacogenetics by reviewing some key fundamental concepts in pharmacology and genetics as they apply to the general discipline of pharmacogenetics. The authors also briefly provide a framework for establishing the role of the clinical laboratory in this process.

0272-2712/08/$ - see front matter © 2008 Elsevier Inc. All rights reserved.
doi:10.1016/j.cll.2008.10.004   *labmed.theclinics.com*

An article prepared by Dr. Weber discusses the history of pharmacogenomics and how advanced technology has transformed pharmacogenetics from a descriptive to a predictive science. This article also provides an extensive literature review of the genetic markers predictive of human drug response. These two introductory articles are followed by three others that discuss applications in anticoagulation, an important area in which much has been written by way of immediate clinical application of PGx testing. The first of these articles, prepared by Drs. Hill and Duncan, provides an overview of PGx in anticoagulation therapy with pertinent clinical scenarios. The second article, prepared by Drs. Lyon, McMillin and Melis, discusses the current status of methods and allele variants relevant for anticoagulation therapy. This article is followed by an overview by Drs. Bon Homme, Reynolds, and Linder that discusses new dynamic pharmacogenetic models in anticoagulation therapy. This group of articles collectively provides an overview on the role of PGx in anticoagulation medicine with contributions currently made and also projected to be available for patient care as PGx is extended with the use of bioinformatics.

Next, the issue provides an overview by Drs. Ageciras-Schmnich, O'Kane, and Snozek of PGx applications in oncology, with examples related to the drug tamoxifen and irinotecan therapies; this article identifies key findings in this area of research. The use of PGx applications in pain management is an exciting area that is gaining much attention. Dr. Webster presents a clear synopsis of the clinical needs and is followed by Drs. Reynolds, Ramey-Hartung, and Jortani, who summarize the value of PGx testing involving 2D6 and OPRM1 as markers for opioid therapy.

The third interesting area for clinical application of PGx is in behavioral disorders. This section begins with an article by Drs. deLeon, Arranz, and Ruano covering clinical laboratory tests that are now available by way of PGx testing modalities that apply to psychiatric disorders. This is followed by a discussion of PGx-guided dose modifications of antidepressants, prepared by Drs. Seeringer and Kirchheiner. The section on behavioral health is concluded by an overview of PGx testing in schizophrenia and posttraumatic stress disorder prepared by Drs. Ramey-Hartung, Reynolds, and El-Mallakh that focuses on several relevant PGx-related biomarkers, including 2D6, DRD2, 5HTT, 5HTR. An important area of medicine–respiratory disorders related to asthma therapy and it relations of PGx testing is discussed by Ms. Yu and Dr. Lewis Bukaveckas.

This compendium of articles in *Clinics in Laboratory Medicine* will be a great tool for researchers thinking about joining the field of PGx, because it covers the major areas of research in the field of PGx and it points out the strengths and weaknesses of this rapidly growing field of clinical medicine. Physicians and other health professionals who want to gain more understanding of this exciting field in the clinical laboratory will also find these articles stimulating. Finally, this selection of articles will be a great tool for students anxious to learn about the science of pharmacogenetics and its various clinical applications.

Kristen K. Reynolds, PhD
PG$_{XL}$ Laboratories
Vice President, Laboratory Operations
201 East Jefferson Street, Suite 309,
Louisville, KY 40202, USA

E-mail address: kreynolds@pgxlab.com

Roland Valdes, Jr, PhD, FACB
Professor and Senior Vice Chairman
Department of Pathology and Laboratory Medicine, and
Professor of Biochemistry and Molecular Biology
University of Louisville School of Medicine
MDR Building, Room 222
511 South Floyd Street
Louisville, KY 40292, USA

E-mail address: rvaldes@louisville.edu

ELSEVIER
SAUNDERS

CLINICS IN
LABORATORY
MEDICINE

Clin Lab Med 28 (2008) 485–497

Fundamentals of Pharmacology and Applications in Pharmacogenetics

Mohammad Al-Ghoul, PhD[a],
Roland Valdes, Jr, PhD, FACB[a,b],*

[a]Department of Pathology and Laboratory Medicine, University of Louisville,
School of Medicine, Louisville, KY, USA
[b]Department of Biochemistry and Molecular Biology, University of Louisville,
School of Medicine, Louisville, KY, USA

This article provides an introduction to the fundamental principles of pharmacokinetics (PK) and pharmacodynamics (PD) as they apply to understanding the application of pharmacogenetics (PGx) in a clinical setting. PGx establishes connections between the disciplines of pharmacology and genetics. As such, one functional component of PGx involves establishing relationships between phenotypes and genotypes with respect to predicting the response of medications in individual patients. The article begins by briefly describing each of the above concepts, followed by a discussion of the clinical utility of pharmacokinetics and pharmacodynamics in a laboratory medicine setting and then relates to the evolving field of PGx from the perspective of clinical laboratory medicine. The practice of laboratory medicine serves as a catalyst for transitioning PGx into clinical settings, and as such the, article concludes with a description of the future role of clinical laboratories in the application of PGx to patient care.

Overview of pharmacology

Pharmacology is the study of drugs and how the function of living tissues and organisms is modified by the effect of drugs and other chemical substances. Historically, knowledge of pharmacologic responses to drugs has been based on average population responses. Recently, however, technology has opened doors toward allowing a more individualized response

* Corresponding author. University of Louisville School of Medicine, Department of Pathology and Laboratory Medicine, MDR Bldg, Room 222, 511 South Floyd Street, Louisville, KY 40292.
  E-mail address: rvaldes@louisville.edu (R. Valdes, Jr).

0272-2712/08/$ - see front matter
doi:10.1016/j.cll.2008.07.001

assessment based on information specific to an individual's biochemistry. This approach has led to the concept that is more personalized medicine relative to drug selection and dosing. Two fundamental principles that hold information relative to individualizing drug response and that drive descriptive pharmacology are pharmacokinetics and pharmacodynamics (Fig. 1) [1]. These concepts are important, because they form the basis for understanding how PGx may lead to a focused personalized medicine approach to clinical pharmacology.

PK involves the relationship describing the effect on drugs by a living organism, including the rates of absorption, distribution, metabolism, and excretion (ADME, see Fig. 1) [1]. Many biological, physiological, and physicochemical factors influence the transfer processes of drugs in the body and thus influence the overall rate and extent of ADME for those drugs. In short, PK involves rates of processing and transport of drugs. Basic principles of PK are used to determine the dose of a drug required to provide the steady-state concentration of the medicine needed to achieve the required therapeutic response. As a result, PK is considered one key element for establishing a rational design of an individualized dosage regimen. The main objectives are to maintain an optimum drug concentration at the receptor site, to produce the desired therapeutic response for a specific period, and to minimize any adverse or toxic effects of the drug.

PD, on the other hand, describes the effect of the drug on the body and is based on the fundamental principles founded on the receptor occupancy theory (see Fig. 1) [1]. PD is driven by the nature of the drug–receptor interaction, which is affected by the number and affinity of receptors, as well as the drug concentration at the receptor site. This underlies the importance of achieving a sustained steady-state effective concentration of drugs in the fluids bathing

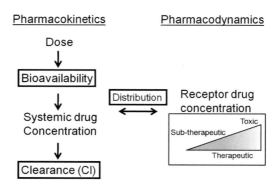

Fig. 1. Overview of pharmacology. Pharmacokinetics (PK) relates to the effect of the body on the drug and principally includes bioavailability, distribution, and clearance. Pharmacodynamics (PD) relates to drug concentration and receptor availability. The response to drug concentrations may be therapeutic, subtherapeutic, or toxic, depending on considerations involving both PK and PD principles. (*From* Linder MW, Valdes R Jr. Pharmacogenetics: fundamentals and applications. Therapeutic drug monitoring and toxicology. AACC 1999;20(1):10; with permission.)

the receptors (eg, blood, cerebrospinal fluid [CSF]) when a sustained drug response is desired. The article then focuses on the role of PK in developing PGx, because most of the information linking genetics to personalized medicine related to dosing of a drug is related to drug metabolism. Subsequent articles in this series also address the receptor-mediated responses and demonstrate how PK and PD are combined to provide valuable clinical information.

Therapeutic drug monitoring (TDM), more recently referred to as therapeutic drug management, involves using measured serum drug concentrations along with PK and PD principles to individualize and optimize a patient's response to drug therapy. The response to drug concentrations may be therapeutic, subtherapeutic, or toxic, and these depend upon considerations involving both PK and PD principles. The aim is to optimize therapeutic response by maintaining serum drug concentrations within a therapeutic range (the concentration at which the drug maximizes effectiveness and minimizes toxicity). TDM is applied most effectively to a small number of drugs with a narrow range of safe and effective serum drug concentrations. Optimum drug treatment is achieved by maintaining those effective concentrations within a population and, better yet, a patient-specific therapeutic range. Fig. 2 shows the relationship between dose rate, PK, serum drug concentration, and pharmacological response [1]. The healthcare provider will determine the dose and frequency of drug administration typically based on the drug's known bioavailability and clearance rate, which will result in steady-state serum concentrations that provide the expected therapeutic response. Examples of drugs that typically are monitored using TDM principles are amikacin, amitriptyline, carbamazepine, cyclosporine, digoxin, gentamicin, imipramine, lidocaine, lithium, methotrexate, nortriptyline, phenytoin, theophylline, tobramycin, valproic acid, and vancomycin, among others.

The balance of drug adsorption, metabolism, distribution, and excretion with dose rate maintains the required steady-state systemic drug concentration [1]. The average steady-state concentration of a drug ($C_{avg\ ss}$) is maintained by dose rate, bioavailability (f), and clearance (Cl) of the drug (see Fig. 2). The catalytic activity of drug metabolizing enzymes (DMEs) is the

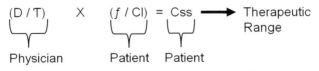

$$(D\,/\,T) \quad X \quad (f\,/\,Cl)\ =\ Css\ \longrightarrow\ \text{Therapeutic Range}$$

Physician   Patient   Patient

D : Dose rate
T : frequency of administration of dose
f : Bioavailability
Cl : Clearance
Css : steady state serum drug concentration

Fig. 2. Dose rate (D) and frequency of dose administration (τ) determined by physician based on the patient bioavailability (f) and clearance (Cl) to accomplish steady-state serum drug concentration. *Abbreviation:* Css, steady state serum drug concentration.

principal determinant of the drug extraction ratio (ER), which is a measure of the fraction of drug cleared from circulation as it passes through whichever organ is involved in its metabolism [1]. The ER is a component of bioavailability and clearance of the drug:

$$f = (\% \text{ Absorption})(1 - \text{ER}) \tag{1}$$

Where % absorption is the fraction of the dose absorbed.

$$\text{Cl} = (q)(\text{ER}) \tag{2}$$

Where q is the blood flow (amount per unit time) to the organ where metabolism occurs.

From the equations 1 and 2, it becomes evident that as the ER is decreased, f increases, and Cl decreases [1]. This explains the concept of how changes in the activity of DMEs alter the steady-state concentration of a drug at a constant dose rate. In essence, the extraction ratio plays a critical role in establishing the steady-state concentration in blood for any given dose of drug.

The theory of receptor occupancy is central to understanding drug action and it is linked to effective concentrations of a drug in blood. The relationship between the blood concentration of a drug and the response caused by that drug is shown in Fig. 3 [2]. Fig. 3A depicts the number of available receptors, and 3B, the affinity of the receptors. Genetic contributions might be responsible for both scenarios. Genetic variants (ie, polymorphisms) in the

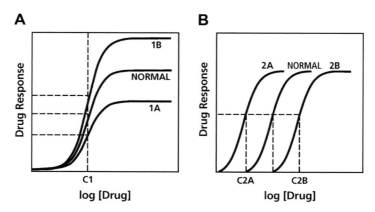

Fig. 3. Pharmacodynamics of drug response. (*A*) Relationship between the number of receptors and drug response, where 1A is a low number, and 1B is a high number of receptors. (*B*) Relationship of drug response to affinity of receptors, where 2A is a high affinity receptor, and 2B is low affinity. The 50% effective drug concentration C2A is lower for a high-affinity receptor compared with concentration C2B. (*From* Weber W. Human drug response. In: Bobrow M, Harper PS, Scriver C, et al, editors. Pharamcogenetics. New York: Oxford University Press; 1997. p. 28; with permission.)

promoter region of a gene responsible for expressing the receptor protein may reduce the number of receptors, whereas, genetic variants in the coding region may affect the affinity of the receptors [3]. A second important relationship is that between the dose of a drug and the subsequent concentration of the drug in blood [3]. The descriptive elements that dictate the concentration–time curve or area under the curve (AUC) of a drug in blood are shown in Fig. 4 [2], including the subsequent action on the target cells and, hence, the link to the importance of receptor-mediated responses.

Cytochrome P450 system and drug metabolism

In relation to pharmacology, cytochrome P450s (CYPs) are a family of heme-containing enzymes that catalyze the conversion of lipophilic substances into hydrophilic molecules that can then be excreted by the kidneys into the urine [3]. They represent a major part of the body's powerful detoxification systems. The CYP system metabolizes endogenous and exogenous substrates through various reactions, including epoxidation, N-dealkylation, O-dealkylation, S-oxidation, hydroxylation, and others [4]. Exogenous substances (products ingested or absorbed) include not only pharmaceutical compounds given as therapeutic drugs, but also foodstuffs, dietary components, occupational pollutants, and industrial chemicals [3]. As a group, the CYP450 enzymes often are referred to as DMEs. The metabolic process generally is described as having two phases, based on the nature of the transformation. Phase 1 involves an oxidative process, whereas phase 2 metabolism is generally conjugative [3]. The CYP mixed-function monooxygenase system is probably the most important element of phase 1 metabolism in

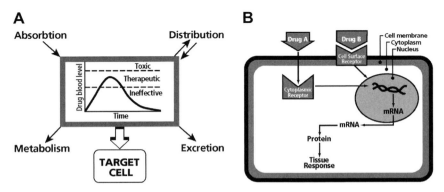

Fig. 4. (A) Area under the curve (AUC) for a drug dose and the elements controlling the shape and magnitude of the curve, typically absorption, distribution, metabolism, and excretion. (B) Interaction of a drug with a cell surface receptor or a cytoplasmic receptor. (*From* Weber W. Human drug response. In: Bobrow M, Harper PS, Scriver C, et al, editors. Pharmacogenetics. New York: Oxford University Press; 1997. p. 22; with permission.)

mammals [5]. Importantly, more than half of all drugs are cleared primarily by the CYP system [3].

The CYP system is a gene family found at multiple chromosome loci, each with tandem arrays of genes, and each gene with substantial polymorphism [3]. This system is an illustration of gene expansion, multigene families, and allelic functional variation. Genomics as a discipline has supplied a rich resource of gene mapping data and the individual variants in each gene at the single nucleotide polymorphism (SNP) and chromosome locus levels. The 57 CYP isoforms now known in people, along with the hundreds of genetic variations, have produced a large set of biomarkers believed to be predictive of susceptibility to specific toxins [3]. The fact that the pharmaceutical industry routinely includes an assessment of the main metabolic pathways of a candidate drug to derive clinical pharmacological correlations is indicative of the importance of this knowledge [3]. Additionally, certain CYP alleles also can be disease susceptibility markers and some are known to be implicated in detoxification or activation of environmental toxins associated with cancer risk [6,7].

The CYP Nomenclature Committee (www.cypalleles.ki.se) has defined the nomenclature used to categorize the variant alleles of the CYP enzyme system. In general, the descriptors rely on the hierarchy of the genetic structures involved in the construction of the enzymes. Fig. 5 describes the common basis for CYP nomenclature [1,8]. Of the CYP enzymes described to date, those most closely related to clinical applications through PGx testing are the 2D6, 2C9, and 2C19 enzymes which play a role in the metabolism of more than 30% of all prescription drugs [9,10]. Factors such as high prevalence of variants in human populations and a wide range of therapeutics metabolized by these enzymes render them among the most relevant DMEs for PGx diagnostics [3].

One important example is the CYP2D6 enzyme system, known to metabolize many of the most widely-prescribed drugs in the United States for depression, cardiovascular disease, schizophrenia, attention deficit–hyperactivity disorder, prevention of nausea and vomiting for patients undergoing cancer chemotherapy, and symptoms of allergies and colds [10–13].

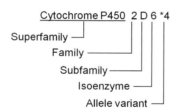

Fig. 5. Nomenclature system for designating enzymes and alleles of cytochrome P450. (*From* Linder MW, Valdes R Jr. Pharmacogenetics: fundamentals and applications. Therapeutic drug monitoring and toxicology. AACC 1999;20(1):11; with permission.)

CYP2D6 polymorphism has differential prevalence and effect among population subgroups. For example, CYP2D6 polymorphisms associated with slow drug metabolism are found in approximately 5% to 10% of Caucasians and 1% to 3% of Hispanics, African Americans, and Asian Americans [10].

Overview of pharmacogenetics

Introduction to genetic concepts in pharmacogenetics

A gene is a linear sequence of nucleotides; these nucleotides are joined together in sequence by means of a phosphodiester bond between the 5' and 3' carbons of the deoxyribose moiety of the nucleotide. Genes consist of a long strand of DNA containing a promoter that controls the activity of a gene and its coding and noncoding sequences. The coding sequence determines what protein the gene produces, while noncoding sequences can regulate the conditions of gene expression. A gene is the basic physical and functional unit of heredity; the proper scientific term for this functional unit is allele. Alleles are forms of the same gene with differences in their sequence of DNA bases. These differences contribute to each person's unique physical features and phenotypes. When a gene contains the proper elements, the coding and noncoding sequences are copied by transcription, producing an mRNA copy of the gene's information [14]. This mRNA then can direct the synthesis of the protein by means of the genetic code [14].

Genetic polymorphism in pharmacogenetics

Genetic polymorphism occurs in the form of gross structural change, including nucleotide substitution, complete gene deletion, gene duplication, and genetic translocation where portions of similar genes are combined creating a new gene hybrid. By far, the most common form of genetic polymorphism is a single nucleotide polymorphism (SNP) where the nucleotide sequence at one specific position is changed by substitution, translocation, insertion, or deletion [7]. Each of these changes in the gene structure introduces a variant form of the gene into the population gene pool and is designated an allele of the original gene [7]. Thus, an allele is an inherited gene that is present in each nucleated cell of the body. Because of the diploid structure of the human genome, each cell carries two copies of each gene. Two copies of the same allele yield a homozygous genotype and any combination of two different alleles yields a heterozygous genotype. A convention for CYP allele nomenclature has been developed (see Fig. 5) [1]. For most CYP genes, where genetic polymorphism has been characterized, the most common sequence and that which is active, is denoted by the gene abbreviation followed by an asterisk and the number 1. This allele then serves as the reference sequence to which all other alleles of that gene are compared [7].

The various types of genetic polymorphism generally can be classified by their resulting influence on protein expression (eg, drug receptor or metabolizing enzyme) or ultimate phenotype. Genetic polymorphism resulting in gene deletion invariably leads to loss of function and no production of the gene product. In contrast, gene duplication and multiduplication most commonly leads to increased expression of the gene product and a hyperactivity phenotype [7]. An exception to this is duplication of an allele that includes additional structural variation leading to loss of function. Genetic translocation typically yields a nonfunctional gene. SNPs can result in various changes in the expressed protein function depending on where the polymorphism occurs in the overall gene structure. SNPs in the 5′ regulatory domain may influence gene regulation [7]. SNPs in the coding exons only influence function if there is a resulting amino acid change that alters the protein function [7]. SNPs within the intron regions are typically silent unless the SNP alters a nucleotide critical for splicing of the RNA during maturation which typically leads to loss or decrease in protein function [7].

Clinical pharmacogenetics

PGx, as demonstrated in Fig. 6, forms the third and base leg of the pharmacology triangle, representing the molecular basis that drives PK and PD [1]. The terms pharmacogenomics and PGx have been used interchangeably and a definition of either remains controversial [15]. PGx generally is regarded as the study or clinical testing of genetic variation that gives rise to differing response to drugs, while pharmacogenomics is the broader application of genomic technologies to new drug discovery [16,17]. Generally, PGx considers one or at most a few genes of interest, while pharmacogenomics considers the entire genome. Based on the FDA E15 Definitions for Genomic Biomarkers, Pharmacogenomics, Pharmacogenetics, Genomic Data, and Sample Coding Categories published in April of 2008, pharmacogenomics is the study of variations of DNA and RNA characteristics as related to drug response. PGx as a subset of genomics is defined as the study

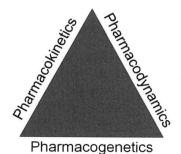

Fig. 6. Pharmacogenetics establishes the functional basis of pharmacokinetics and pharmacodynamics. (*From* Linder MW, Valdes R Jr. Pharmacogenetics: fundamentals and applications. Therapeutic drug monitoring and toxicology. AACC 1999;20(1):9; with permission.)

of variations in DNA sequence as related to drug response. In any event, PGx represents the relationship between gene-based markers and pharmacology as it relates to the processing or function of drugs. The clinical utility of PGx is embodied principally in the ability to predict either the most appropriate dosing of a medicine (usually based on metabolic information) or the selection of a particular medicine for a given individual (usually based on metabolism or receptor status). This expectation has led to the concept of a personalized medicine approach to drug therapeutics. Although the science and clinical application of PGx seem to be converging rapidly, the clinical application to patient care is not a common practice as yet.

As a general rule, PGx links differences in drug metabolism and response (phenotype) with differences in gene structure (genetic polymorphism) [18]. Most alleles encoding DMEs reside within a somatic chromosome and thus are inherited in a nonsex-linked Mendelian fashion [18]. On the basis of observed phenotyping data, such as metabolic ratios of drug components in blood and urine, a reasonable separation can be demonstrated between extensive metabolizers (normal metabolizers), rapid metabolizers (generally referred to as ultrarapid), and poor metabolizers in their ability to biotransform specific medications. Currently, relative to metabolism, the patient phenotype based on his/her genotype is defined as extensive, intermediate, poor, or ultraextensive metabolizers. The differences between these phenotypes are explained in Box 1 [19]. This nomenclature recently has been challenged as not being sufficiently descriptive and requiring modification [3].

Current and future applications of pharmacogenetics

Pharmacogenetics and health needs

It is anticipated that, once the applications of PGx diagnostics become more fully realized, they may address certain major health needs, including reducing adverse drug reactions (ADRs). ADRs have been reported to be the result of nearly 3 million incorrect or ineffective drugs prescriptions annually [10]. PGx testing holds promise to help physicians prescribe drugs and dosages in ways that are more likely to fit individual patient responses and thus, reduce the number of ADRs [10,20]. Although some resistance and controversy still exist, PGx also may help to improve the productivity of new drug pipelines [10,21]. The use of PGx in clinical trial design and patient accrual could lead to reductions in the time needed to develop a drug-from 10 to 12 years to perhaps as little as 3 to 5 years [10]. The ability to stratify patient groups using genomic biomarkers should enable discernment of significant treatment or causative effects that otherwise would have been diluted in more heterogeneous populations. In addition to these applications, and from a pharmacotherapeutic perspective, the use of PGx information may enable development of drugs tailored for patients who have rare or orphan conditions and other underserved patient groups [10,21].

Box 1. Phenotypic categories as determined by pharmacogenetic testing for cytochrome P450 enzymes

Ultraextensive metabolizers (UM)—may require an increased dosage because of higher than normal rates of drug metabolism. Simultaneously treating with medication that inhibits metabolization also has proven effective. Genotypes consistent with UM phenotype include three or more active genes producing the drug- metabolizing enzyme and therefore have increased metabolic capacity.

Extensive metabolizers (EM)—represent the norm for metabolic capacity. Genotypes consistent with the EM phenotype include two active forms of the gene producing the drug-metabolizing enzyme and therefore possess the full complement of drug metabolizing capacity. Generally, extensive metabolizers can be administered drugs, which are substrates of the enzyme following standard dosing practices.

Intermediate metabolizers (IM)—may require lower than average drug dosages for optimal therapeutic response. In addition, multiple drug therapy should be monitored closely.

Poor metabolizers (PM)—are at increased risk of drug-induced adverse effects because of diminished drug elimination (accumulation) or lack of therapeutic effect resulting from failure to generate the active form of the drug. Genotypes consistent with the PM phenotype are those with no active genes producing the drug- metabolizing enzyme. These individuals have a deficiency in drug metabolism.

This information helps healthcare providers with powerful information to adjust a patient's drug dose.

Data from Valdes R Jr, Payne D, Linder M, et al. Guidelines and recommendations for laboratory analysis and application of pharmacogenetics in clinical practice. Available at: http://www.aacc.org/members/nacb/LMPG/OnlineGuide/DraftGuidelines/Pharmacogenetics/Pages/default.aspx. National Academy of Biochemistry, in press.

PGx also has the potential to improve treatments for chronic diseases which pose the greatest morbidity and cost burden for the United States and other developed nations. Application of PGx to disease prognosis may help reduce costs by curtailing the duration of illness through more effective treatments and minimizing the costs associated with ineffective treatment and avoidable ADRs or appropriate response to prolonged drug therapy. One example of this is the drug tamoxifen [22] used to treat breast cancer. Tamoxifen is an inactive prodrug that must be metabolized by CYP2D6 into its more potent metabolite, endoxifen, in order to elicit its effect therefore, understanding a patient's CYP2D6 metabolic status is crucial to the success of tamoxifen therapy. A subsequent article in this issue will address the issues and utility of tamoxifen PGx in detail (see article by Algeciras-Schimnich and colleagues, elsewhere in this issue). A growing body of PGx knowledge involves interindividual genetic variations that result in variation in drug transporters, DMEs, and drug targets, all contributing to differences in how people respond to the same medications. For example, a genetic basis for aspirin resistance has been postulated to exist, although published studies from which to draw conclusions have been limited. Goodman and colleagues [23] published a systemic review of all candidate gene association studies in aspirin resistance. They searched electronic databases through December 2007 for all studies investigating any candidate gene for aspirin resistance in people. Their data support a possible genetic association between the polymorphism in the GPIIIa platelet receptor (PIA/A2) and aspirin resistance in healthy subjects, with the effect diminishing in the presence of cardiovascular disease. Further studies are needed in this area of research. One limitation for these studies is the technique used to measure and define aspirin resistance, since investigators have yet to decide on standardized techniques.

Although most of the current attention to PGx focuses on a small number of recent molecular breakthroughs, much of the potential health benefit of PGx resides in some of the longer-standing, more widely used products. Indeed, most ADRs, including many that are likely to be influenced by genotype, arise with use of older drugs. Much existing information on PGx for guiding available therapies appears to be ignored. A recent review of package insert information for the top 200 drugs prescribed in 2003 found that PGx data were available in the literature for 71.3% of these drugs, but that such information appeared in the package inserts of only a few of these drugs. Much of the valuable information about PGx that is available remains to be put to use [10].

The clinical laboratory and pharmacogenetics

The clinical laboratory is the principal vehicle for providing PGx testing services to the medical community [24]. These services include providing access to testing, selecting appropriate testing profiles and, among other responsibilities, providing the evidence required to formulate decisions on medical applications [24]. The use of gene-based information to stratify patients, preferably before they are prescribed medication, is perceived as having substantial merit to the practice of laboratory medicine. For PGx to find its way into general clinical practice, however, methods must be established for translating the genetic information provided by the marker (eg, SNP variants in genes for metabolic enzymes or receptors) into a quantifiable and reliable altered dosing or drug selection scheme. Controversy remains about the interpretation and reporting of PGx information. Several reports, however, provide valuable examples of the interpretation and reporting of PGx. Linder and colleagues [25] proposed dosing schemes for warfarin by modeling the question of what modifications to current dosing schemes may be most appropriate for individuals who have an impairment in warfarin metabolism. Currently, clinical pharmacogenomics is being pursued actively, with the expectation that the future of PGx in the clinical laboratory is still in its infancy but has enormous possibilities [26–28].

Acknowledgment

We thank Ms. Rosemary Williams for her help in the editing of this manuscript.

References

[1] Linder MW, Valdes R Jr. Fundamentals of pharmacogenetics. In: Wong SHY, Linder MW, Valdes R Jr, editors. Pharmacogenomics and proteomics: enabling the practice of personalized medicine. AACC Press; 2006. p. 13–9.

[2] Weber W. Human drug response. In: Bobrow M, Harper PS, Scriver C, et al, editors. Pharmacogenetics. New York: Oxford University Press; 1997. p. 21–40.

[3] Valdes R Jr, Payne D, Linder M, et al. Guidelines and recommendations for laboratory analysis and application of pharmacogenetics in clinical practice. Available at: http://www.aacc.org/members/nacb/LMPG/OnlineGuide/DraftGuidelines/Pharmacogenetics/Pages/default.aspx. National Academy of Clinical Biochemistry 2007, in press.

[4] Wilkinson GR. Drug metabolism and variability among patients in drug response. N Engl J Med 2005;352(21):2211–21.

[5] de Leon J, Armstrong SC, Cozza KL. Clinical guidelines for psychiatrists for the use of pharmacogenetic testing for CYP450 2D6 and CYP450 2C19. Psychosomatics 2006;47(1):75–85.

[6] Feigelson HS, McKean-Cowdin R, Coetzee GA, et al. Building a multigenic model of breast cancer susceptibility: CYP17 and HSD17B1 are two important candidates. Cancer Res 2001; 61(2):785–9.

[7] Linder MW, Valdes R Jr. Genetic mechanisms for variability in drug response and toxicity. J Anal Toxicol 2001;25(5):405–13.

[8] Nelson DR, Kamataki T, Waxman DJ, et al. The P450 superfamily: update on new sequences, gene mapping, accession numbers, early trivial names of enzymes, and nomenclature. DNA Cell Biol 1993;12(1):1–51.

[9] Phillips KA, Van Bebber SL. Measuring the value of pharmacogenomics. Nat Rev Drug Discov 2005;4(6):500–9.

[10] Tuckson RV. Realizing the promise of pharmacogenomics: opportunities and challenges. Biotechnology Law Report 2007;26(3):261–91.

[11] Johnson JA, Cavallari LH. Cardiovascular pharmacogenomics. Exp Physiol 2005;90(3): 283–9.

[12] Johnson JA, Humma LM. Pharmacogenetics of cardiovascular drugs. Brief Funct Genomic Proteomic 2002;1(1):66–79.

[13] Agundez JA, Gallardo L, Ledesma MC, et al. Functionally active duplications of the CYP2D6 gene are more prevalent among larynx and lung cancer patients. Oncology 2001; 61(1):59–63.

[14] Gerstein MB, Bruce C, Rozowsky JS, et al. What is a gene, post-ENCODE? History and updated definition. Genome Res 2007;17(6):669–81.

[15] Khoury MJ. Genetics and genomics in practice: the continuum from genetic disease to genetic information in health and disease. Genet Med 2003;5(4):261–8.
[16] Sikka R, Magauran B, Ulrich A, et al. Bench to bedside: pharmacogenomics, adverse drug interactions, and the cytochrome P450 system. Acad Emerg Med 2005;12(12):1227–35.
[17] Weinshilboum R, Wang L. Pharmacogenomics: bench to bedside. Nat Rev Drug Discov 2004;3(9):739–48.
[18] Linder MW, Valdes R Jr. Fundamentals and applications of pharmacogenetics for the clinical laboratory. Ann Clin Lab Sci 1999;29(2):140–9.
[19] Linder MW, Prough RA, Valdes R Jr. Pharmacogenetics: a laboratory tool for optimizing therapeutic efficiency. Clin Chem 1997;43(2):254–66.
[20] Hopkins MM, Ibarreta D, Gaisser S, et al. Putting pharmacogenetics into practice. Nat Biotechnol 2006;24(4):403–10.
[21] Schmedders M, van Aken J, Feuerstein G, et al. Individualized pharmacogenetic therapy: a critical analysis. Community Genet 2003;6(2):114–9.
[22] Goetz MP, Kamal A, Ames MM. Tamoxifen pharmacogenomics: the role of CYP2D6 as a predictor of drug response. Clin Pharmacol Ther 2008;83(1):160–6.
[23] Goodman T, Ferro A, Sharma P. Pharmacogenetics of aspirin resistance: a comprehensive systematic review. Br J Clin Pharmacol 2008;66(2):222–32.
[24] Linder MW, Valdes R Jr. Pharmacogenetics in the practice of laboratory medicine. Mol Diagn 1999;4(4):365–79.
[25] Linder MW, Looney S, Adams JE 3rd, et al. Warfarin dose adjustments based on CYP2C9 genetic polymorphisms. J Thromb Thrombolysis 2002;14(3):227–32.
[26] Valdes R Jr, Linder MW. Fine-tuning pharmacogenetics: paradigm for linking laboratory results to clinical action. Clin Chem 2004;50(9):1498–9.
[27] Valdes R Jr, Linder MW, Jortani SA. What is next in pharmacogenomics? Translating it to clinical practice. Pharmacogenomics 2003;4(4):499–505.
[28] Linder MW, Valdes R Jr. Pharmacogenetics: fundamentals and applications. Therapeutic drug monitoring and toxicology. Washington (DC):AACC 1999;20(1):9–17.

ELSEVIER
SAUNDERS

CLINICS IN
LABORATORY
MEDICINE

Clin Lab Med 28 (2008) 499–511

Pharmacogenetics: From Description to Prediction

Wendell W. Weber, MD, PhD

Department of Pharmacology, University of Michigan Medical School, 1301BMSRB III, 1150 West Medical Center Drive, Ann Arbor, MI 48109-5632, USA

Pharmacogenetics has reached a point at which many of the complexities of human drug response and disease are understood and some can be predicted. Genomics and computational tools, combined with an extensive record of research in cells of individuals and in model systems that define the field, have fueled the transformation of pharmacogenetics from a descriptive to a predictive science.

As new tools develop and discovery continues, many facets of biologic systems are just coming into view. The biologic landscape will continue to change rapidly for the foreseeable future and beyond, delivering new insights that must be accommodated as our understanding of the genomics of human drug response advances. As a consequence of these changes, we often hear "pharmacogenetics" and "pharmacogenomics" used interchangeably but, whichever term is used, the main problem is how best to accommodate the shift in the scale of operations entailed in going from genetics to genomics. Like most other fields of biology, pharmacogenetics is primarily data driven, without which, attempts at prediction would likely fail.

Before 1950, little was known about the specifics of heredity on human drug response, but during the years in and around both 1950 and 2000, remarkable advances were made in the quest for knowledge about heredity. Because of the singular nature of events capping these two periods (the discovery of the DNA double helix and the maturation of the human genome initiative), earlier discoveries that led to the emergence of modern pharmacology and genetics were overshadowed. For an account of those earlier events, we turn to the middle of the nineteenth century, whence the foundations of pharmacogenetics stretching from its beginnings to the present can be divided into four periods (Box 1). The first of these periods defines the

E-mail address: wwweber@umich.edu

doi:10.1016/j.cll.2008.05.002   *labmed.theclinics.com*

Box 1. Foundation of pharmacogenetics

1850 to 1910: Cellular foundations
Mendel's laws discovered, lost, and rediscovered
Biotransformation of chemicals discovered in humans
Drug receptors inferred
Chromosomes defined as locus of heredity
Chemical individuality of man defined

1910 to 1960s: Molecular foundations
DNA identified as the hereditary material
DNA double helix described
Central dogma of molecular biology formulated
Protein polymorphism established
Human chromosomes enumerated
Disease associated with chromosomal aberrations
Experimental pharmacogenetics emerges

1960s to date: Informational foundations
DNA-RNA hybrid helix discovered
Genetic code for nuclear genes determined
Readout of nuclear genes worked out
Recombinant DNA technologies invented
Mitochondrial genome sequence determined
Mitochondrial genetic code determined
Polymerase chanin reaction invented
Genomics tools developed
DNA polymorphisms identified
Human genome initiative started
Epigenetics modifies gene expression

1990s to date: Genomics foundations
Large-scale, high-throughput techniques developed
Maturation of the human genome initiative
Toxicogenomics applied to drug discovery
Construction of risk profiles for drug susceptibility
    (www.hapmap.org)
Epigenomics

---

cellular foundations of early pharmacology and genetics, whereas the second defines the molecular foundations of modern genetics and pharmacology; the informational and genomic foundations of modern biology and pharmacogenetics are defined by the last two periods [1].

The timeline in Fig. 1 shows the emergence of experimental pharmacogenetics in the 1950s and the start-up of recombinant DNA technologies with

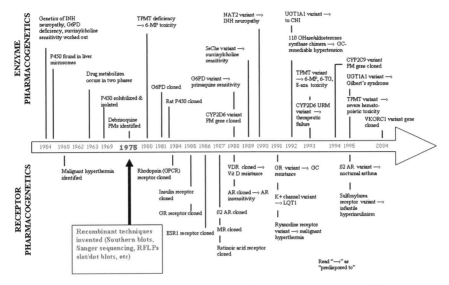

Fig. 1. Benchmarks in human enzyme and receptor pharmacogenetics.

the invention of Southern blots in 1975; it also shows the growth of the field throughout the 1980s, foreshadowing trends toward genomics in and around the 1990s. As the invention and development of new genomics tools have continued, the informational period overlaps the genomics era, and both extend to the present.

From its emergence in the 1950s, the primary goal of experimental pharmacogenetics has been to understand how genetic variation in molecular processes in cells is linked to human drug responses. Initially, and subsequently for almost 3 decades, analysis of biochemical and physiologic genetic variation was the primary source of understanding these processes. But the widespread adoption of newly invented methods for sequencing the genome, and for identifying and locating genomic lesions of medical importance that began in the 1970s, marked the beginning of a period that has completely transformed life science research, including that of pharmacogenetics. By drawing on specific examples of genetic markers predictive of human drug response, and genetic markers predictive of outcomes and therapeutic benefits in cancer, the following discussion intends to show that the field of pharmacogenetics has moved from an earlier descriptive phase to that of a predictive science. Currently, clinical application of many genetic markers is limited by lack of knowledge about the effects of modifying genes on these markers, by lack of knowledge about their prevalence and risk contribution in different ethnogeographic populations, and by fragmentary information about how genetic factors interact with physiologic or pathologic and other environmental factors. Establishing the relationship of genotype to phenotype is thus a major challenge [2,3].

Genetic markers predictive of human drug response

Polymorphic genes that encode the drug-metabolizing enzymes, transporters, drug receptors, and other proteins can serve as valuable markers predictive of the efficacy and adverse responses in human subjects. Several examples of these genetically polymorphic markers are listed in Table 1 [4–40]. These proteins determine the disposition and elimination of, and the response to, most drugs; they often occur at high frequencies in human subjects. They have been used extensively, particularly those that are members of the drug-metabolizing enzymes, to characterize the genetics and molecular basis of normal and genetically altered drug responses and to document the diversity of different raciogeographic populations.

Fig. 1 shows that genetic variation is associated with polymorphisms of many drug-metabolizing enzymes (pharmacokinetic variability). These polymorphic enzymes make up most of the examples tabulated because they preceded the identification of receptor polymorphisms (pharmacodynamic variability) by nearly 3 decades; it follows that the identification of the drug-metabolizing enzyme polymorphisms was almost entirely responsible for guiding the initial development of pharmacogenetics. And because recombinant DNA technologies were not invented before 1975, it is evident that before that date, investigators were almost entirely dependent on human pedigree analysis and other classic genetic methods to characterize the polymorphic traits associated with the drug-metabolizing enzymes. It is also evident from Fig. 1 that the molecular features of receptors (and transporters) were not defined until the mid-1980s, when the recombinant DNA technologies were adopted by many laboratories around the world. Hence, while the pharmacogenetics of drug-metabolizing enzymes moved ahead apace, progress in receptor and transporter pharmacogenetics was delayed for nearly 3 decades.

Because of this lag and because the investigation of receptors and transporters is inherently more difficult, fewer well-studied examples of the latter genetic markers are available. Only two of the markers cited in Table 1, CCR5 and Her-2, are receptors, and one, SLCO1B1, is a transporter. In 2002, Hirschhorn and coworkers [41] reported 268 genes that contain polymorphisms that account for 603 different gene-disease associations. Among these, 166 associations were based on three separate publications, and of these, only 6 associations were highly consistently reproducible (significant in at least 75% of positive studies). Among these 6 associations, 3 were relevant to pharmacogenetics: that for Factor V Leiden, for the CCR5 receptor, and for APOE4 protein. Only 1 of these, that for the CCR5 receptor, directly concerns receptor pharmacogenetics.

In 2008, Katz and colleagues [42] extended the search for associations of greater pharmacogenetic interest, although they limited their study to associations with pharmacokinetic variation. They identified consistently replicated associations for at least one drug between gene variants and human pharmacokinetics for 16 genetically polymorphic proteins. Table 1 provides a selected list of these well-studied proteins, many of which have been known for some time; the table does not include four drug-metabolizing enzymes (ADH4, CYP2A6, CYP2B6, CYP3A5) listed by Katz and colleagues.

The potential that pharmacogenomics offers physicians in adapting drug treatments to the characteristics of individual variants leading to safer and more effective prescribing and dosing is discussed at length in the Winter 2008 issue of the Food and Drug Administration (FDA) *Drug Safety Newsletter* [6]. A link to a table of valid genomic biomarkers in the context of approved drug labels that are currently part of FDA-approved drug labels is included there. The FDA recognizes many of the biomarkers listed in Table 1 as valid for safer, more effective prescribing. The Drug Safety Newsletter also contains links to clinical applications of pharmacogenomics, detection of drug resistance in viruses, and the FDA's role in pharmacogenomics and personalized medicine [6].

Genetic markers predictive of outcomes and therapeutic benefits in cancer

Patients who have cancer in the same stage of disease can have markedly different treatment responses and overall outcomes. Attempts to identify molecular profiles of distinct tumor types by gene expression began in the mid-1990s. In 1996, DeRisi and colleagues [43] were among the first to suggest that DNA microarrays be used to identify several alterations in the expression of genes specific to a tumorogenic phenotype and they demonstrated this point in a melanoma cell line. In 1999, Golub and coworkers [44] set out to develop a systematic, analytic approach to class prediction using the same technology to distinguish acute leukemia types whose histologic appearance was highly similar. Having demonstrated the feasibility of cancer classification based solely on gene expression monitoring, they suggested a general strategy for discovering and predicting cancer classes for other types of cancer, independent of previous biologic knowledge.

Shortly after Golub's report, and using microarray technology, several investigative groups reported progress in predicting outcomes and benefits in cancer treatment [45–51]. Breast cancer, for example, the most common cancer among women and the second leading cause of cancer-related deaths of women in the United States (http://www.cancer.org [breast cancer facts and figures]), illustrates the approaches taken and the progress made. Hedenfalk and coworkers [45] used an approach similar to that of Golub and colleagues to obtain distinctive molecular signatures left by *BRCA1* and *BRCA2* genes in patients who had breast cancer. They demonstrated that significantly different groups of genes are expressed among *BRCA1* mutation-positive tumors, *BRCA2* mutation-positive tumors, and sporadic tumors. van't Veer and associates [46] identified a "poor prognosis" signature strongly predictive of distant metastases in patients who had breast cancer without tumor cells in local lymph nodes; in addition, they identified

Table 1
Selected genetic markers consistently predictive of efficacious and adverse drug responses

Genetic marker response	Clinical indication	Prediction	Selected references
CYP2C9 and warfarin	Prevention and treatment of thrombotic disease	Variant alleles predispose to reduced warfarin requirements (warfarin sensitivity).	[4–7]
VKORC1 and warfarin		Variant alleles predispose to increased warfarin requirements (warfarin resistance) and reduced warfarin requirements.	
CYP2C19 and PPIs	Reduction of gastric acidity	Variant alleles (extensive metabolizers) are predisposed to variation in response to PPIs such as omeprazole, lansoprazole, and pantoprazole.	[8,9]
CYP2D6[a] and codeine	Treatment of mild pain	Poor metabolizers fail to respond to codeine. Ultrarapid metabolizers exhibit exaggerated responses to codeine.	[10–13]
CYP2D6[a] and tamoxifen	Treatment of breast cancer	Poor metabolizer women are predisposed to higher recurrence rates of breast cancer because they produce lower levels of anticancer tamoxifen metabolite, endoxifen. Women taking tamoxifen should avoid taking drugs (eg, SSRIs) that inhibit CYP2D6. SSRIs such as venlafaxine are preferred treatment of hot flashes because they do not inhibit CYP2D6; paroxetine and fluoxetine should be avoided because they are potent inhibitors of CYP2D6.	[15]
UGT1A1 and irinotecan	Treatment of colorectal cancer (in 5-fluorouracil refractory patients)	Persons who harbor the variant promoter allele UGT1A1*28 are predisposed to severe grades of irinotecan-induced diarrhea and neutropenia. The UGT1A1/UGT1A7 SNP appears to be a superior risk predictor.	[16–18,14]
Dihydropyrimidine dehydrogenase and 5-fluorouracil	Treatment of cancers of the gastrointestinal tract, breast, and head and neck	Persons harboring a G→A point mutation are predisposed to severe fluorouracil-induced toxicity.	[19,20]

TPMT and antileukemic/ immune drugs	Treatment of leukemia and immune disorders	Persons harboring TPMT-deficient alleles are predisposed to serious acute and delayed intolerance to thiopurine immunosuppressive and antileukemic drugs. They are also predisposed to interactions with agents that are potent TPMT inhibitors (olsalazine). They may also be predisposed to cefazolin-induced hypoprothrombinemia.	[21–24]
Mitochondrial ALDH2 and alcohol (ethanol)	Not applicable	Persons harboring the defective ALDH2 Glu487Lys variant allele are predisposed to aversive facial flushing and acute vasomotor dilation to ethanol; as a result of this aversive reaction, they drink significantly less alcohol and are highly protected from alcoholism.	[25–27]
ADH2 and ethanol	Not applicable	ADH2 contains an Arg>His polymorphism at codon 47. Persons harboring the ADH2 Arg allele are predisposed to heavy ethanol drinker status and habitual drinking; the effect of drinking behavior is significant, regardless of the presence of the ALDH2 Glu487Lys polymorphism.	[27]
FMO3 and fish odor syndrome	Not applicable	Persons harboring FMO3 variants are predisposed to exude the odor of rotting fish in sweat, breath, and urine on eating foods that yield trimethylamine as a breakdown product. Affected persons suffer devastating educational, economic, and social consequences.	[28,29]
Factor V Leiden and susceptibility to deep vein thrombosis	Not applicable	Persons harboring Factor V Leiden are predisposed to deep vein thrombosis, especially at younger ages, during pregnancy, and during the puerperium. Persons who harbor the mutant coagulant protein may never suffer thrombosis, but may be lifelong candidates for anticoagulant therapy. Carriers of factor V Leiden combined with G20210A prothrombin SNP have increased risk for thrombosis after the first episode.	[30,31]

(continued on next page)

Table 1 (*continued*)

Genetic marker response	Clinical indication	Prediction	Selected references
CCR5 and susceptibility to HIV-1 infection	Not applicable	Adult homozygotes for CCR5Δ32 are highly protected from HIV infection; progression of the disease is slowed in adult heterozygotes. Another receptor allele, CCR2-641, plays a protective role in mother-to-infant transmission and delays HIV-1 progression after infection.	[32–35]
Herceptin-2 and trastuzumab	Treatment of HER2-dependent breast cancer	The humanized monoclonal antibody, trastuzumab, in combination with appropriate adjuvant chemotherapy, significantly slows progression and improves survival of women affected by HER2-dependent metastatic breast cancer.	[36,37]
OATP-C, SLCO1B1, and bile acids, sulfates and glucuronide conjugates, plus many drug substrates, including pravastatin, methotrexate, and rifampin	Not applicable	The reduced activity of novel allele of OATP-C gene called OATP-C*15 contains N130D and V174A SNPs; various carriers of the functionally deficient OATP-C*15 variants exhibit reduced liver uptake of rifampin and possibly reduced capacity for rifampin-mediated induction of liver drug-metabolizing enzymes and transporters.	[38–40]

Abbreviations: ADH2, alcohol dehydrogenase 2; ALDH2, aldehyde dehydrogenase 2; CCR, chemokine receptor; CYP, cytochrome P450; FMO3, flavin monooxygenase 3; HER2, human epidermal growth factor receptor 2; OATP-C, organic anion transporting polypeptide C; PPIs, proton pump inhibitors; SLCO1B1, solute carrier organic anion transporter family, member 1B1; SNP, single nucleotide polymorphism; SSRIs, selective serotonin reuptake inhibitors; TPMT, thiopurine methyltransferase; UGT, UDP-glucuronosyltransferase; VKORC1, vitamin K oxidoreductase complex 1.

[a] At least 25% of all prescribed drugs are estimated to be subject to metabolism by CYP2D6 polymorphic alleles.

a signature for tumors of *BRCA1* carriers. van't Veer and colleagues provided a tool to tailor adjuvant systemic therapy that could greatly decrease the risk for adverse side effects and health care expenditure. A study by van de Vijver and coworkers [47] described a gene expression signature as a predictor for breast cancer survival among patients younger than 53 years of age who had either stage I or II disease. The gene signature was a powerful predictor of outcome among younger patients, and it indicated that the prognosis profile might be a useful guide to adjuvant therapy in patients who have lymph node–positive cancer. Liu and colleagues [51], on examining the prognostic role of gene signatures, identified an "invasive gene signature" (IGS) in patients who had breast cancer, and found a significant association between IGS and overall and metastasis-free survival. This genetic signature was also associated with the prognosis in medulloblastoma, lung cancer, and prostate cancer. The IGS was more strongly predictive of clinical outcomes when combined with the "wound response" signature (a 512-gene signature that correlates with overall survival and metastasis-free survival in patients who have breast cancer).

Despite advances in understanding genetic and molecular pathways that are altered in cancerous cells, investigators believed that diagnosis and treatment would benefit from a more quantitative approach to decision making. In 2004, Paik and colleagues [52] resolved some important issues by developing an assay to predict recurrence in patients who have tamoxifen-treated, node-negative breast cancer, to determine a risk group (low, intermediate, high) for each patient; the recurrence score (RS) was validated in a large clinical trial. In an extension of this work, Paik and colleagues [53] examined the relationship of the RS to benefit from chemotherapy. Patients who had high-RS tumors benefited greatly from chemotherapy, whereas patients who had low-RS tumors derived minimal, if any, benefit. Patients who had intermediate-RS tumors did not appear to benefit from chemotherapy, but the uncertainty of the estimate did not exclude a clinically important benefit. The RS assay, which is commercially available, not only quantified the likelihood of breast cancer occurrence but also predicted the magnitude of the chemotherapy benefit.

A further advance is reported by Yu and colleagues [54] who used gene expression profiling of estrogen-receptor–positive breast cancer cells to screen for a robust estrogen-regulated gene signature that might serve as a better indicator of cancer outcome. These investigators identified 532 estrogen-induced genes and further developed a 73-gene signature that best separated 286 primary breast cancers into prognostic subtypes. This signature separated patients who had received endocrine therapy into two prognostic subgroups suggesting tumor hormonal sensitivity. The 73-gene signature provides predictive value for patient survival, independent of other clinical parameters and outperforms previously reported molecular outcome signatures.

Many of the studies performed in support of molecular profiling of human cancers are retrospective, and it appears the field is poised to begin its next phase, the conduct of prospective trials of adjuvant chemotherapy in patients who have various forms of early cancer [55]. For breast cancer, the next phase has already begun, with retrospective data indicating that adjuvant treatment is beneficial in patients who have high-risk breast tumors [53]. Next, cancer genomics will probably emphasize three areas: molecular profiles associated with response or resistance to targeted therapies, clinical trials based on molecular profiles that indicate beneficial effects from targeted therapies, and evaluation of the significance of epigenetic phenomena (DNA methylation, histone modification) in cancer genomics. Several signaling pathways are associated with sensitivity or resistance to agents targeting these pathways. In lung cancer, one of the best examples concerns epidermal growth factor receptor (EGFR) mutations and amplification that identify patients who have small cell lung cancers who respond to EGFR tyrosine kinase inhibitors. Given the approval of the EGFR inhibitor, erlotinib, and the angiogenesis inhibitor, bevacizumab, for treatment of lung cancer, it is important to create molecular tools to predict the response of these cancers to single agents or combination chemotherapies. The signature reported by Chen and colleagues [56] includes ERRB3, a gene associated with sensitivity to EGFR tyrosine kinase inhibitors. Additional examples of molecular markers of resistance include expression of excision repair cross-complementation group1 gene (ERCC1) (resistance to cisplatin-based adjuvant therapy) and ras mutations (resistance to cisplatin-based therapy and EGFR tyrosine kinase inhibitors) [55]. It is expected that treatment of individual patients who have early-stage cancers will be targeted on the basis of the molecular characteristics of the tumors.

Summary

Many of the complexities of human drug response are sufficiently well understood to transform the field of pharmacogenetics from a descriptive to a predictive science. Clinical application of these markers is currently limited by lack of knowledge about the effects of modifying genes, about their prevalence and risk contribution in different ethnogeographic populations, and by fragmentary information about how genetic factors interact with physiologic or pathologic and other environmental factors. Nevertheless, progress has been notable, as exemplified in the identification of genetic markers predictive of pharmacokinetic variation, and in markers predictive of outcome and therapeutic benefit in the treatment of cancer.

References

[1] Weber WW. Pharmacogenetics. 2nd edition. New York: Oxford University Press, 2008.
[2] Peltonen L, McKusick VA. Genomics and medicine. Dissecting human disease in the post-genomic era. Science 2001;291(5507):1224–9.

[3] Feero WG, Guttmacher AE, Collins FS. The genome gets personal—almost. JAMA 2008; 299(11):1351–2.

[4] Rettie AE, Tai G. The pharmocogenomics of warfarin: closing in on personalized medicine. Mol Interv 2006;6(4):223–7.

[5] Flockhart DA, O'Kane D, Williams MS, et al. Pharmacogenetic testing of CYP2C9 and VKORC1 alleles for warfarin. Genet Med 2008;10(2):139–50.

[6] Feature article: Pharmacogenomics. 2008. Ref Type: Internet Communication.

[7] Gage BF, Lesko LJ. Pharmacogenetics of warfarin: regulatory, scientific, and clinical issues. J Thromb Thrombolysis 2008;25(1):45–51.

[8] Desta Z, Zhao X, Shin JG, et al. Clinical significance of the cytochrome P450 2C19 genetic polymorphism. Clin Pharmacokinet 2002;41(12):913–58.

[9] Andersson T, Flockhart DA, Goldstein DB, et al. Drug-metabolizing enzymes: evidence for clinical utility of pharmacogenomic tests. Clin Pharmacol Ther 2005;78(6):559–81.

[10] Sindrup SH, Brosen K. [Combination preparations of codeine and paracetamol]. Ugeskr Laeger 1998;160(4):448–9 [in Danish].

[11] Dalen P, Frengell C, Dahl ML, et al. Quick onset of severe abdominal pain after codeine in an ultrarapid metabolizer of debrisoquine. Ther Drug Monit 1997;19(5):543–4.

[12] Gasche Y, Daali Y, Fathi M, et al. Codeine intoxication associated with ultrarapid CYP2D6 metabolism. N Engl J Med 2004;351(27):2827–31.

[13] Koren G, Cairns J, Chitayat D, et al. Pharmacogenetics of morphine poisoning in a breastfed neonate of a codeine-prescribed mother. Lancet 2006;368(9536):704.

[14] Innocenti F, Undevia SD, Iyer L, et al. Genetic variants in the UDP-glucuronosyltransferase 1A1 gene predict the risk of severe neutropenia of irinotecan. J Clin Oncol 2004;22(8):1382–8.

[15] Hayes DF, Stearns V, Rae J, et al. A model citizen? Is tamoxifen more effective than the aromatase inhibitors if we pick the right patients? J Natl Cancer Inst 2008;100:610–3.

[16] Iyer L, Das S, Janisch L, et al. UGT1A1*28 polymorphism as a determinant of irinotecan disposition and toxicity. Pharmacogenomics J 2002;2(1):43–7.

[17] Lankisch TO, Schulz C, Zwingers T, et al. Gilbert's syndrome and irinotecan toxicity: combination with UDP-glucuronosyltransferase 1A7 variants increases risk. Cancer Epidemiol Biomarkers Prev 2008;17(3):695–701.

[18] Hoskins JM, Marcuello E, Altes A, et al. Irinotecan pharmacogenetics: influence of pharmacodynamic genes. Clin Cancer Res 2008;14(6):1788–96.

[19] Van Kuilenburg AB, Muller EW, Haasjes J, et al. Lethal outcome of a patient with a complete dihydropyrimidine dehydrogenase (DPD) deficiency after administration of 5-fluorouracil: frequency of the common IVS14+1G > A mutation causing DPD deficiency. Clin Cancer Res 2001;7(5):1149–53.

[20] Van Kuilenburg AB, Meinsma R, Zoetekouw L, et al. High prevalence of the IVS14 + 1G > A mutation in the dihydropyrimidine dehydrogenase gene of patients with severe 5-fluorouracil-associated toxicity. Pharmacogenetics 2002;12(7):555–8.

[21] McLeod HL, Krynetski EY, Relling MV, et al. Genetic polymorphism of thiopurine methyltransferase and its clinical relevance for childhood acute lymphoblastic leukemia. Leukemia 2000;14(4):567–72.

[22] Weinshilboum R. Thiopurine pharmacogenetics: clinical and molecular studies of thiopurine methyltransferase. Drug Metab Dispos 2001;29(4 Pt 2):601–5.

[23] Lewis LD, Benin A, Szumlanski CL, et al. Olsalazine and 6-mercaptopurine-related bone marrow suppression: a possible drug-drug interaction. Clin Pharmacol Ther 1997;62(4): 464–75.

[24] Wood TC, Johnson KL, Naylor S, et al. Cefazolin administration and 2-methyl-1,3,4-thiadiazole-5-thiol in human tissue: possible relationship to hypoprothrombinemia. Drug Metab Dispos 2002;30(10):1123–8.

[25] Higuchi S, MUramatsu T, Shigemori K, et al. The relationship between low Km aldehyde dehydrogenase phenotype and drinking behavior in Japanese. J Stud Alcohol 1992;53(2): 170–5.

[26] Crabb DW, Edenberg HJ, Bosron WF, et al. Genotypes for aldehyde dehydrogenase deficiency and alcohol sensitivity. The inactive ALDH2(2) allele is dominant. J Clin Invest 1989;83(1):314–6.

[27] Matsuo K, Wakai K, Hirose K, et al. Alcohol dehydrogenase 2 His47Arg polymorphism influences drinking habit independently of aldehyde dehydrogenase 2 Glu487Lys polymorphism: analysis of 2,299 Japanese subjects. Cancer Epidemiol Biomarkers Prev 2006;15(5): 1009–13.

[28] Dolphin CT, Janmohamed A, Smith RL, et al. Missense mutation in flavin-containing mono-oxygenase 3 gene, FMO3, underlies fish-odour syndrome. Nat Genet 1997;17(4): 491–4.

[29] Treacy EP, Akerman BR, Chow LM, et al. Mutations of the flavin-containing monooxygenase gene (FMO3) cause trimethylaminuria, a defect in detoxication. Hum Mol Genet 1998; 7(5):839–45.

[30] Ridker PM, Hennekens CH, Lindpaintner K, et al. Mutation in the gene coding for coagulation factor V and the risk of myocardial infarction, stroke, and venous thrombosis in apparently healthy men. N Engl J Med 1995;332(14):912–7.

[31] De Stefano V, Martinelli I, Mannucci P, et al. The risk of recurrent deep venous thrombosis among heterozygous carriers of both factor V Leiden and the G20210A prothrombin mutation. N Engl J Med 1999;341:801–6.

[32] Liu R, Paxton WA, Choe S, et al. Homozygous defect in HIV-1 coreceptor accounts for resistance of some multiply-exposed individuals to HIV-1 infection. Cell 1996;86(3):367–77.

[33] Samson M, Libert F, Doranz BJ, et al. Resistance to HIV-1 infection in Caucasian individuals bearing mutant alleles of the CCR-5 chemokine receptor gene. Nature 1996;382(6593): 722–5.

[34] Dean M, Carrington M, Winkler C, et al. Genetic restriction of HIV-1 infection and progression to AIDS by a deletion allele of the CKR5 structural gene. Hemophilia Growth and Development Study, Multicenter AIDS Cohort Study, Multicenter Hemophilia Cohort Study, San Francisco City Cohort, ALIVE Study. Science 1996;273(5283):1856–62.

[35] Mangano A, Kopka J, Batalla M, et al. Protective effect of CCR2-64I and not of CCR5-delta32 and SDF1-3'A in pediatric HIV-1 infection. J Acquir Immune Defic Syndr 2000; 23(1):52–7.

[36] Slamon DJ, Leyland-Jones B, Shak S, et al. Use of chemotherapy plus a monoclonal antibody against HER2 for metastatic breast cancer that overexpresses HER2. N Engl J Med 2001;344(11):783–92.

[37] Hudis CA. Trastuzumab-mechanism of action and use in clinical practice. N Engl J Med 2007;357(1):39–51.

[38] Tirona RG, Leake BF, Wolkoff AW, et al. Human organic anion transporting polypeptide-C (SLC21A6) is a major determinant of rifampin-mediated pregnane X receptor activation. J Pharmacol Exp Ther 2003;304(1):223–8.

[39] Tamai I, Nezu J, Uchino H, et al. Molecular identification and characterization of novel members of the human organic anion transporter (OATP) family. Biochem Biophys Res Commun 2000;273(1):251–60.

[40] Katz DA, Carr R, Grimm DR, et al. Organic anion transporting polypeptide 1B1 activity classified by SLCO1B1 genotype influences atrasentan pharmacokinetics. Clin Pharmacol Ther 2006;79(3):186–96.

[41] Hirschhorn JN, Lohmueller K, Byrne E, et al. A comprehensive review of genetic association studies. Genet Med 2002;4(2):45–61.

[42] Katz DA, Murray B, Bhathena A, et al. Defining drug disposition determinants: a pharmacogenetic–pharmacokinetic strategy. Nat Rev Drug Discov 2008;7(4):293–305.

[43] DeRisi J, Penland L, Brown PO, et al. Use of a cDNA microarray to analyse gene expression patterns in human cancer. Nat Genet. 1996;14:457–60.

[44] Golub TR, Slonim DK, Tamayo P, et al. Molecular classification of cancer: class discovery and class prediction by gene expression monitoring. Science 1999;286(5439):531–7.

[45] Hedenfalk I, Duggan D, Chen Y, et al. Gene-expression profiles in hereditary breast cancer. N Engl J Med 2001;344(8):539–48.

[46] van't Veer LJ, Dai H, van de Vijver MJ, et al. Gene expression profiling predicts clinical-outcome of breast cancer. Nature 2002;415(6871):530–6.

[47] van de Vijver MJ, He YD, van't Veer LJ, et al. A gene-expression signature as a predictor of survival in breast cancer. N Engl J Med 2002;347(25):1999–2009.

[48] Bild AH, Yao G, Chang JT, et al. Oncogenic pathway signatures in human cancers as a guide to targeted therapies. Nature 2006;439(7074):353–7.

[49] Bild AH, Potti A, Nevins JR. Linking oncogenic pathways with therapeutic opportunities. Nat Rev Cancer 2006;6(9):735–41.

[50] Fan C, Oh DS, Wessels L, et al. Concordance among gene-expression-based predictors for breast cancer. N Engl J Med 2006;355(6):560–9.

[51] Liu R, Wang X, Chen GY, et al. The prognostic role of a gene signature from tumorigenic breast-cancer cells. N Engl J Med 2007;356(3):217–26.

[52] Paik S, Shak S, Tang G, et al. A multigene assay to predict recurrence of tamoxifen-treated, node-negative breast cancer. N Engl J Med 2004;351(27):2817–26.

[53] Paik S, Tang G, Shak S, et al. Gene expression and benefit of chemotherapy in women with node-negative, estrogen receptor-positive breast cancer. J Clin Oncol 2006;24(23):3726–34.

[54] Yu J, Yu J, Cordero KE, et al. A transcriptional fingerprint of estrogen in human breast cancer predicts patient survival. Neoplasia 2008;10(1):79–88.

[55] Herbst RS, Lippman SM. Molecular signatures of lung cancer—toward personalized therapy. N Engl J Med 2007;356(1):76–8.

[56] Chen HY, Yu SL, Chen CH, et al. A five-gene signature and clinical outcome in non-small-cell lung cancer. N Engl J Med 2007;356(1):11–20.

ELSEVIER
SAUNDERS

CLINICS IN
LABORATORY
MEDICINE

Clin Lab Med 28 (2008) 513–524

Overview of Pharmacogenetics in Anticoagulation Therapy

Charles E. Hill, MD, PhD[a,b,*],
Alexander Duncan, MD[a,c]

[a]Department of Pathology and Laboratory Medicine, Emory University School of Medicine,
Emory University Hospital, 1364 Clifton Road, Atlanta, GA 30322, USA
[b]Molecular Diagnostics Laboratory, Emory University School of Medicine, Atlanta, GA, USA
[c]Special Coagulation Laboratory, Emory University School of Medicine, Atlanta, GA, USA

Although interest has grown significantly in personalizing medical treatment, the greatest potential benefit for customized drug dosing should be realized for drugs with narrow therapeutic indices or profound toxicity profiles. A great deal of effort has been devoted to studying the pharmacogenetics of warfarin therapy because of the difficulties in dosing and the substantial morbidities/mortalities associated with under- and overtreatment. However, controversy still exists about whether pharmacogenetic testing is useful for all patients and cost-effective. Clinical implementation of warfarin pharmacogenetic testing has been challenging, and incorporation of this information into dosing regimens has been slow. Although many challenges exist to widespread adoption of pharmacogenetic-based dosing of warfarin, the personalization of warfarin therapy has great potential.

Karl Paul Link [1] from the University of Wisconsin investigated the compounds in spoiled sweet clover, trying to elucidate the causes of hemorrhage in cattle after ingestion. The offending compound isolated in his laboratory was named *dicoumarol* and used in medical care as an anticoagulant for many years. Subsequent to their synthesis of dicoumarol, scientists in Link's laboratory synthesized many similar compounds, including one believed too toxic to use. Mark Stahmann, with the help of the Wisconsin Alumni Research Foundation (WARF), patented the compound that would later be named *warfarin* (US Patent #2,427,578) [1].

---

* Corresponding author. Department of Pathology and Laboratory Medicine, Emory University School of Medicine, Emory University Hospital, 1364 Clifton Road, Room F147A, Atlanta, GA 30322, USA.
  E-mail address: cehill@emory.edu (C.E. Hill).

0272-2712/08/$ - see front matter © 2008 Elsevier Inc. All rights reserved.
doi:10.1016/j.cll.2008.09.002
labmed.theclinics.com

Although warfarin's anticoagulant properties have been known for many years, its mechanism of action has only recently been fully elucidated. It was clear in the earliest use of coumarins that dicumarol had similar structure to vitamin K [2]. These compounds have been collectively referred to as vitamin K antagonists based on competition studies and structural similarities, even though the intracellular target had not been identified. Recently, vitamin K epoxide reductase complex subunit 1 (VKORC1) was identified as the intracellular target for warfarin [3]. Vitamin K epoxide is a necessary cofactor in the gamma carboxylation of clotting factors II,VII, IX, and XI and proteins C and S. Inhibition of VKORC1 results in decreased levels of activated clotting factors and thereby reduces the efficiency with which blood clots [4].

Metabolism of warfarin

Vitamin K is a necessary cofactor in the synthesis of several coagulation factors in the liver. These "vitamin K–dependent coagulation factors" are gamma carboxylated by gamma glutamyl carboxylase. Through inhibiting this activity, coagulation factors II, VII, IX, and X along with protein C and S are synthesized at a substantially reduced rate [4]. Vitamin K is typically recycled after the gamma carboxylation reaction. The resulting vitamin K epoxide is reduced to vitamin K hydroquinone in two steps, both catalyzed by vitamin K epoxide reductase [5]. Vitamin K hydroquinone is necessary for activity of gamma glutamyl carboxylase. Dietary vitamin K may enter the cycle through an NADPH-dependent reduction, bypassing VKORC1.

In 2005, the gene responsible for multiple coagulation factor deficiency type II was identified through positional cloning [6]. The vitamin K epoxide reductase complex subunit 1 gene encodes an integral membrane protein, which is part of a multiprotein complex responsible for the recycling of reduced vitamin K from vitamin K epoxide. These findings made it clear that the intracellular target for warfarin is VKORC1. Warfarin acts to inhibit VKORC1, leading to decreased levels of reduced vitamin K. Reduced vitamin K is a necessary cofactor in the gamma carboxylation of coagulation factors II, VII, IX, and X, and proteins C and S. Because inhibition of VKORC1 decreases the amount of these coagulation factors, the ability of blood to clot is reduced but not completely eliminated.

Warfarin, as administered, is a racemic mixture of R- and S-warfarin. The bioavailability of warfarin is excellent and approaches 100% [7,8]. Warfarin is primarily protein-bound and therefore seems to have a relatively low volume of distribution [7,9]. Although R-warfarin does have anticoagulant properties, the anticoagulant activity of S-warfarin is significantly greater than the R enantiomer [7,8]. S-warfarin is cleared by hydroxylation catalyzed by cytochrome P450 2C9 (CYP2C9), yielding inactive metabolites that are excreted in the urine. R-warfarin is cleared more slowly by a different series of P450 isozymes [8].

CYP2C9 is a member of the cytochrome P450 family of enzymes and is responsible for the clearance of approximately 20% of commercially available pharmaceuticals. Several substrates, inhibitors, and inducers have been characterized. Originally described as the enzyme responsible for the hydroxylation of phenytoin [10], much more research has been devoted to studying its role in the clearance of warfarin. The crystal structure of CYP2C9 with warfarin bound has been solved [11], and thus, the amino acids involved in forming the binding pocket for warfarin have been identified. Therefore, variations in amino acid composition unsurprisingly have an impact on the metabolic activity of this enzyme.

Warfarin efficacy is currently monitored with functional assays [12,13]. Patients on warfarin have a prothrombin time (PT) measured frequently, usually at least every 2 weeks. The corrected PT, or international normalized ratio (INR), is used to determine if the patient is taking a sub- or supratherapeutic dose of warfarin. INR testing is often performed more frequently in patients being initiated on warfarin or those with very labile INRs. The INR has been used for many years and is a good marker of anticoagulation status. However, high INRs do not directly indicate that patients will have a bleeding event and low INRs do not necessarily predict thrombosis [14,15].

CYP2C9 polymorphisms

Genetic variations in the CYP2C9 gene have been identified that alter the rate of hydroxylation by this enzyme [16–18]. These genetic polymorphisms are widely distributed and vary by region and ethnicity. The effects of these changes are not readily apparent to patients and no phenotype associated with these polymorphisms is easily discernable. The first indication of a polymorphism may be the overactivity or poor clearance of a standard drug dose for a drug metabolized by this enzyme.

Although the P450 Nomenclature Committee [18] currently recognizes 30 alleles for CYP2C9, only the *1, *2, and *3 alleles have been well studied with regard to warfarin. By convention, the most common allele is designated *1. The proteins encoded by *2 and *3 alleles have reduced activity compared with the protein produced by the *1 allele. In vitro data indicate that, compared with the *1 allele, the *2 and *3 alleles produce CYP2C9 proteins with 70% and 20% activity, respectively [19–21]. These alleles are defined by specific single nucleotide polymorphisms (SNPs) in exons 3 and 7, respectively, and are differentially distributed within the population [22–25]. The *2 allele is present in approximately 10% to 12% of Caucasians in the United States and Europe and very rare in Africans and African Americans. Alleles other than *1 are extraordinarily uncommon in Asian populations. The *3 allele is less common, present in 8% of Caucasians and virtually nonexistent in Africans or African Americans.

Both the *2 and *3 alleles are associated with lower maintenance warfarin dose; however, the effects of each allele differ [23,26–29]. Meta-analysis of several studies has estimated that the *2 allele is responsible for a 17% reduction in maintenance dose, whereas the *3 allele accounts for a 37% dose reduction [23]. In homozygous form, these alleles have a much greater impact, with typical doses reduced by 50% to 75% compared with patients who have the homozygous *1. Compound heterozygotes have also been identified and seem to be similar to homozygous poor metabolizers (*2 or *3).

As with all P450 enzymes, enzyme activities have wide variability among individuals who have the same genotype [30]. These genes are inducible and clear many different compounds. Diet, medications, and vitamin supplementation can create significant differences in warfarin clearance, even within a group sharing the same genotype.

Since most P450 activity resides within the gut and liver, the health of these organs is a critical determinant of warfarin clearance. Patients who have significant liver disease may require much lower or much higher doses than patients who have normal liver function. Because the P450 system is inducible, predicting the exact dosing changes necessitated by liver disease is very difficult. It is also becoming apparent that an increasing proportion of patients who underwent liver transplantation are being prescribed warfarin. Although transplantation improves liver function, it adds a level of variability to drug clearance, which is not easily quantified. Recent experience in the authors' institution has led to a realization that, in at least some cases, transplants occur across genotypes for CYP2C9 and VKORC1. Although the specific impact of these transplants has not been studied, in the authors' experience the genotype of the donor (rather than the recipient) is likely responsible for the phenotype demonstrated after transplantation. Poor metabolizer status in the donor liver may be exaggerated by the low-level injury resulting from the trauma of transplantation and the polypharmacy to reduce the risk for rejection.

Although poorly studied, some evidence shows that the CYP2C9*5 and *6 alleles may be of importance to warfarin clearance [24]. Using losartan as an in vivo test of CYP2C9 activity, patients who had the *5 allele were found to have impaired losartan oxidation compared with patients who had the *1; however, the number of patients who had variant genotypes was small. In vitro data support that *5, *6, *8, and *11 alleles all have reduced activity compared with *1. The clinical relevance of these changes has not been determined.

Although clearance of S-warfarin by CYP2C9 is an important determinant of interindividual dosing variability, many other factors have been implicated in maintenance dose. Clearly, the amount of vitamin K in the diet has a substantial impact on both inter- and intraindividual dosing [30]. Diet may also account for clearance differences observed in different ethnic groups. Although the factors resulting in the observed differences have not been elucidated, clearance of warfarin was seen to be different between

Caucasian and Japanese populations, even for persons who had homozygous *1 alleles [31].

Multiple SNPs have also been identified within the noncoding regions of the *VKORC1* gene [32–34]. These may be used to define multiple haplotypes; however, many of these SNPs cosegregate and therefore can be grouped [32]. These haplotypes can be grouped into types A and B, wherein patients who have type A haplotypes have been found to have lower maintenance doses of warfarin than those who have type B haplotypes. Subsequently, defining the haplotypes by either the −1639 SNP (−1639 G>A) or the 1173 intronic SNP (1173 C>T) has become more commonplace. It is now clear that the A haplotype (−1639 A and 1173 T) results in decreased mRNA levels for *VKORC1* and thereby lower expression of the protein. Therefore, it is best to consider CYP2C9 variants as poor metabolizers (pharmacokinetic) and VKOR variants as having decreased levels of target, thereby altering stoichiometry (pharmacodynamic).

VKORC1 accounts for a greater proportion of interindividual variability compared with CYP2C9. The geographic and ethnic distributions of VKORC1 variants do not mirror those for CYP2C9 [32–34]. Approximately 37% of Caucasians carry at least one low-dose allele for VKORC1. In contrast, the low-dose allele is homozygous in approximately 90% of Asian patients, whereas CYP2C9 variants represent a vanishingly small percentage.

Slightly more than 50% of the interindividual dosing variability of warfarin can be accounted for by typical pharmacologic parameters, such as body weight (or surface area), age, CYP2C9 genotype, and VKORC1 genotype [35–38]. Other genes participate in this pathway that likely contribute to dosing variability in only small amounts [39–41]. Currently, SNPs in gamma glutamyl carboxylase, calumenin, and Apo E are not believed to have significant impact on the dosing variability of warfarin. Vitamin K levels are difficult to assess in real-time, but might have a substantial impact on the level of anticoagulation because exogenous vitamin K enters the vitamin K cycle independent of VKORC1. These factors are not currently well studied. Temporal changes in vitamin K intake are associated with labile INRs and may lead to frequent dose adjustments.

Clinical implementation

Many clinicians currently use the dosing initiation schemes recommended by the American College of Chest Physicians or the British Committee for Standards in Haematology [12,13]. Both groups recommended conservative dosing while initiating warfarin therapy. Typical schemes involve a starting dose of 3 to 5 mg/d for the first 2 to 5 days, followed by dosing adjustments based on the INR. Although not commonly used, a 10-mg dose has been used in some patients who experience a therapeutic INR 1 to 2 days sooner than lower-dose schemes. Typically, the INR measured on day three is used to adjust the dosing of warfarin. Neither recommendation includes physical factors such as weight or body surface area as criteria for selecting initial dose.

Patients older than 60 years are typically started on lower doses (2–5 mg/d) of warfarin [12,13]. Several studies have shown that patients older than 60 years require lower maintenance dose of warfarin and that there is a trend toward lower doses with increasing age [12]. A study of tolerability of warfarin during the first year of therapy showed that major hemorrhage rates are higher in patients aged 80 years or older (13.08 per 100 person-years versus 4.75 for those younger than 80 years) [42]. Many factors have been hypothesized to account for the reduced dose requirement with age. The net result is that older patients are treated very conservatively or do not receive warfarin at all.

The INR is the most commonly used means of assessing the level of anti-coagulation [12,13]. To arrive at an INR, the PT is measured and then normalized using the reference clotting time for the testing laboratory and factor to normalize for the variations in reagents (International Sensitivity Index [ISI]). This process allows a better comparison between patients and laboratories, because the INR should be independent of the reagents used and the laboratory performing the test.

Other means of estimating the in vivo effects of warfarin have been attempted. Direct measurement of warfarin using a limited sampling strategy can predict the area under curve for S-warfarin [43]. However, poor metabolizers were excluded from this study, and therefore applicability to warfarin dosing has not been established. Measurement of circulating vitamin K levels might also be useful in determining the amount of drug necessary to inhibit VKORC1. Although circulating vitamin K levels might yield some information regarding anticoagulation, the intracellular concentration of vitamin K relative to the amount of VKORC1 (and the amount of warfarin) would seem to be the more important measure.

Algorithms using genetic data to predict warfarin dosing have been developed and tested for accuracy [35–38]. These systems use regression models to predict dose based on demographic data, such as age and weight, along with the number of CYP2C9 *2 and *3 alleles and the number of VKORC1 variants. Predicting the maintenance dose before initiation of therapy may allow some of the bleeding events to be eliminated in patients who are poor metabolizers. This hypothesis has not been rigorously tested and is the source of some controversy [44,45].

These dosing models use complex calculations that may prevent widespread adoption by clinicians. To facilitate the estimates, an Internet-based calculator has been implemented [46]. This system is not only capable of predicted final dose but also can be used to refine dosing once the first few INR measurements have been taken. Additionally, a software-based system has been developed that can model the pharmacokinetics of individual patients given their genotypes and INR measurements [47]. This system attempts to use these data to provide dosing attempting to get the INR into the desired therapeutic range as quickly as possible. Many patients have been entered into these systems and extensively tested. However, large clinical trials of these algorithms and tools have not been completed.

Challenges

Clearly, warfarin is underused in populations shown to benefit by randomized controlled clinical trials [42,48–50]. Studies have been undertaken to identify the reasons for underprescribing or early cessation of warfarin treatment. The reasons most commonly cited by prescribing physicians for not initiating warfarin are hemorrhage, falls, previous inability to tolerate warfarin, and patient refusal or nonadherence to therapeutic regimen.

Studies of bleeding risk have predominantly been cohort studies, and the definitions of significant bleeding events have varied. Reported rates for bleeding requiring transfusion, hospitalization, or surgery range from 0.4% to 2.0% per year. Additionally, more adverse bleeding events occur seems to occur in the first 6 weeks of therapy. Patients who have at least one variant allele were at greater risk for a bleeding event during the first 90 days of therapy, with a hazard ratio of 3.94 [42]. When considering patients who have experienced stable dosing, those who have a variant allele are still at increased risk for a bleeding event.

These factors also contribute to the tendency to underanticoagulate. In an outpatient setting, typical therapeutic INRs may be achieved only 50% of the time [51]. When out of the therapeutic range, patients are subtherapeutic more frequently than supratherapeutic. This trend is independent of whether the patients carry variant alleles at CYP2C9 or VKORC1. This cautious approach may explain why patients who have variant alleles also have a longer time to stable dosing compared with those who have *1 homozygous alleles.

Although retrospective analysis indicates that patients who have *2 and *3 alleles are at greater risk for an adverse event, very few reports show a reduction in the incidence of adverse events or time to stable INR if genotype-based dosing is used [52,53]. However, these studies are small and do not provide sufficient evidence to justify universal prewarfarin genotyping. For these reasons, most health care centers have not yet adopted genotypic dosing. Studies are currently underway to determine if using genotype-based dosing during the initial phase of warfarin therapy will reduce adverse events or time to therapeutic levels.

Implementation of prospective genotype-based dosing depends on timely acquisition of accurate genotype data [54]. The genotype data must be generated quickly if it is to be used prospectively to determine the starting dose. Although technologic advances have made these tests simpler to perform, they still qualify as high-complexity tests. Generally, warfarin is not given acutely. For genetic data to potentially impact length-of-stay, testing must be performed rapidly and on-demand. Currently, four warfarin genotyping assays are cleared by the FDA. Because of the need to extract genomic DNA from a sample, most testing is performed in specialized molecular diagnostic laboratories. In many centers, these laboratories are not staffed 24 hours per day and 7 days per week. Therefore, it may not always be possible to produce genotype results quickly for all patients. The American College of Medical Genetics has issued a policy statement regarding CYP2C9 and VKORC1 genotyping [55]. The group falls short of recommending routine testing, but states that testing may be warranted in specific circumstances. Clinical and regulatory issues must be addressed as pharmacogenetic testing is implemented [56].

In the authors' experience, the greatest current usefulness for pharmacogenetic testing is in patients who have very labile INRs and those who have very low maintenance dose requirements. These patients benefit from more careful monitoring of diet and drug interactions and more frequent outpatient visits to the anticoagulation management clinic. Testing also seems to improve compliance in these patients. When the stigma of "doing something wrong" in the warfarin regimen is removed, patients seem to be more careful of drug dosing and interaction, and experience much less frustration with their warfarin management.

Typically, the greatest barrier to adoption of genotype-based warfarin therapy is physician education. Many clinicians consider genotype data confusing and unnecessary. Patients have been managed for many years without this information, and therefore it is not clear to most practitioners how this new information can be used to improve patient care. Even when a clinician determines that knowing the patient's genotype might help guide dosing, testing is frequently not requested early enough to be used to predict warfarin sensitivity and the first few doses. Although most efforts have been dedicated to predicting maintenance warfarin dose, new algorithms are currently in development using pharmacogenetic data to help refine dosing after patients have started taking warfarin [57,58].

If pharmacogenetics is to be widely used to guide warfarin therapy, evidence must show that the cost of testing has a positive impact on outcome and reduces healthcare costs, at least incrementally. No prospective studies show that the cost of testing is justified by a reduction in length of stay or reduced cost of treating the adverse events. A financial model of the possible impact of pharmacogenetic testing for warfarin has been published by the AEI- Brookings Joint Center for Regulatory Issues [59]. Estimates from this model state that 85,000 serious bleeding events and 17,000 strokes could be avoided each year by using pharmacogenetic testing. The amount of health care cost savings attributed to using genotype-based therapy is between $100 million and $2 billion annually. However, the study has been criticized for the assumptions about how many bleeding events could be prevented [45].

Although very difficult to quantify, overanticoagulation is a major source of litigation for large health care centers. Many health care centers are interested in testing to improve outcomes and reduce financial risk; however, prospective trials must be completed to provide the evidence that pharmacogenetic-based dosing is cost-effective.

Summary

Pharmacogenetic-based drug dosing has the potential to bring individualized therapy to the practice of medicine. The most compelling genetic-drug relationship is between CYP2C9/VKORC1 and warfarin. Algorithms are available to predict maintenance warfarin dose using typical demographic and pharmacogenetic data. However, substantial hurdles to routine testing still exist, including a lack of prospective cost–benefit data and a lack of education for clinicians on how to use the information. In the coming years, this will be only one of many examples of how pharmacogenetics makes personalized medicine possible.

References

[1] Kresge N, Simoni RD, Hill RL. Hemorrhagic sweet clover disease, dicoumarol, and warfarin: the work of Karl Paul Link. J Biol Chem 2005;280(8):e5–6.
[2] Whitlon DS, Sadowski JA, Suttie JW. Mechanism of coumarin action: significance of vitamin K epoxide reductase inhibition. Biochemistry 1978;17(8):1371–7.
[3] Li T, Chang CY, Jin DY, et al. Identification of the gene for vitamin K epoxide reductase. Nature 2004;427(6974):541–4.
[4] Hirsh J, Dalen J, Anderson DR, et al. Oral anticoagulants: mechanism of action, clinical effectiveness, and optimal therapeutic range. Chest 2001;119(Suppl 1):8S–21S.
[5] Fasco MJ, Hildebrandt EF, Suttie JW. Evidence that warfarin anticoagulant action involves two distinct reductase activities. J Biol Chem 1982;257(19):11210–2.
[6] Rost S, Fregin A, Ivaskevicius V, et al. Mutations in VKORC1 cause warfarin resistance and multiple coagulation factor deficiency type 2. Nature 2004;427(6974):537–41.
[7] Wittkowsky AK. Warfarin and other coumarin derivatives: pharmacokinetics, pharmacodynamics, and drug interactions. Semin Vasc Med 2003;3(3):221–30.
[8] Hewick DS, McEwen J. Plasma half-lives, plasma metabolites and anticoagulant efficacies of the enantiomers of warfarin in man. J Pharm Pharmacol 1973;25(6):458–65.
[9] Otagiri M, Maruyama T, Imai T, et al. A comparative study of the interaction of warfarin with human alpha 1-acid glycoprotein and human albumin. J Pharm Pharmacol 1987; 39(6):416–20.
[10] Gut J, Meier UT, Catin T, et al. Mephenytoin-type polymorphism of drug oxidation: purification and characterization of a human liver cytochrome P-450 isozyme catalyzing microsomal mephenytoin hydroxylation. Biochim Biophys Acta 1986;884(3):435–47.
[11] Williams PA, Cosme J, Ward A, et al. Crystal structure of human cytochrome P450 2C9 with bound warfarin. Nature 2003;424(6947):464–8.
[12] Ansell J, Hirsh J, Hylek E, et al. Pharmacology and management of the vitamin K antagonists: American college of chest physicians evidence-based clinical practice guidelines (8th edition). Chest 2008;133(Suppl 6):160S–98S.
[13] Baglin TP, Keeling DM, Watson HG, et al. Guidelines on oral anticoagulation (warfarin) 3rd edition–2005 update. Br J Haematol 2006;132(3):277–85.
[14] Hylek EM, Singer DE. Risk factors for intracranial hemorrhage in outpatients taking warfarin. Ann Intern Med 1994;120(11):897–902.

[15] D'Angelo A, Della Valle P, Crippa L, et al. Relationship between international normalized ratio values, vitamin K-dependent clotting factor levels and in vivo prothrombin activation during the early and steady phases of oral anticoagulant treatment. Haematologica 2002; 87(10):1074–80.

[16] Lee CR, Goldstein JA, Pieper JA. Cytochrome P450 2C9 polymorphisms: a comprehensive review of the in-vitro and human data. Pharmacogenetics 2002;12(3):251–63.

[17] Rettie AE, Jones JP. Clinical and toxicological relevance of CYP2C9: drug-drug interactions and pharmacogenetics. Annu Rev Pharmacol Toxicol 2005;45:477–94.

[18] Allele nomenclature for Cytochrome P450 enzymes. Available at: http://www.cypalleles. ki.se. 2008. Accessed March 28, 2008.

[19] Crespi CL, Miller VP. The R144C change in the CYP2C9*2 allele alters interaction of the cytochrome P450 with NADPH:cytochrome P450 oxidoreductase. Pharmacogenetics 1997;7(3):203–10.

[20] Takanashi K, Tainaka H, Kobayashi K, et al. CYP2C9 Ile359 and Leu359 variants: enzyme kinetic study with seven substrates. Pharmacogenetics 2000;10(2):95–104.

[21] Sullivan-Klose TH, Ghanayem BI, Bell DA, et al. The role of the CYP2C9-Leu359 allelic variant in the tolbutamide polymorphism. Pharmacogenetics 1996;6(4):341–9.

[22] Kirchheiner J, Brockmöller J. Clinical consequences of cytochrome P450 2C9 polymorphisms. Clin Pharmacol Ther 2005;77(1):1–16.

[23] Sanderson S, Emery J, Higgins J. CYP2C9 gene variants, drug dose, and bleeding risk in warfarin-treated patients: a HuGEnet systematic review and meta-analysis. Genet Med 2005;7(2):97–104.

[24] Allabi AC, Gala JL, Horsmans Y, et al. Functional impact of CYP2C9*5, CYP2C9*6, CYP2C9*8, and CYP2C9*11 in vivo among black Africans. Clin Pharmacol Ther 2004; 76(2):113–8.

[25] Scordo MG, Aklillu E, Yasar U, et al. Genetic polymorphism of cytochrome P450 2C9 in a Caucasian and a black African population. Br J Clin Pharmacol 2001;52(4):447–50.

[26] Aithal GP, Day CP, Kesteven PJ, et al. Association of polymorphisms in the cytochrome P450 CYP2C9 with warfarin dose requirement and risk of bleeding complications. Lancet 1999;353(9154):717–9.

[27] Taube J, Halsall D, Baglin T. Influence of cytochrome P-450 CYP2C9 polymorphisms on warfarin sensitivity and risk of over-anticoagulation in patients on long-term treatment. Blood 2000;96(5):1816–9.

[28] Tabrizi AR, Zehnbauer BA, Borecki IB, et al. The frequency and effects of cytochrome P450 (CYP) 2C9 polymorphisms in patients receiving warfarin. J Am Coll Surg 2002;194(3): 267–73.

[29] Margaglione M, Colaizzo D, D'Andrea G, et al. Genetic modulation of oral anticoagulation with warfarin. Thromb Haemost 2000;84(5):775–8.

[30] D'Andrea G, D'Ambrosio R, Margaglione M. Oral anticoagulants: pharmacogenetics relationship between genetic and non-genetic factors. Blood Rev 2008;22(3):127–40.

[31] Takahashi H, Wilkinson GR, Caraco Y, et al. Population differences in S-warfarin metabolism between CYP2C9 genotype-matched Caucasian and Japanese patients. Clin Pharmacol Ther 2003;73(3):253–63.

[32] Rieder MJ, Reiner AP, Gage BF, et al. Effect of VKORC1 haplotypes on transcriptional regulation and warfarin dose. N Engl J Med 2005;352(22):2285–93.

[33] D'Andrea G, D'Ambrosio RL, Di Perna P, et al. A polymorphism in the VKORC1 gene is associated with an interindividual variability in the dose-anticoagulant effect of warfarin. Blood 2005;105(2):645–9.

[34] Reitsma PH, van der Heijden JF, Groot AP, et al. A C1173T dimorphism in the VKORC1 gene determines coumarin sensitivity and bleeding risk. PLoS Med 2005;2(10):e312, 996–998.

[35] Gage BF, Eby C, Milligan PE, et al. Use of pharmacogenetics and clinical factors to predict the maintenance dose of warfarin. Thromb Haemost 2004;91(1):87–94.

[36] Sconce EA, Khan TI, Wynne HA, et al. The impact of CYP2C9 and VKORC1 genetic poly-morphism and patient characteristics upon warfarin dose requirements: proposal for a new dosing regimen. Blood 2005;106(7):2329–33.

[37] Zhu Y, Shennan M, Reynolds KK, et al. Estimation of warfarin maintenance dose based on VKORC1 (-1639 G > A) and CYP2C9 genotypes. Clin Chem 2007;53(7):1199–205.

[38] Gage BF, Eby C, Johnson JA, et al. Use of pharmacogenetic and clinical factors to predict the therapeutic dose of warfarin. Clin Pharmacol Ther 2008;84(3):326–31.

[39] Vecsler M, Loebstein R, Almog S, et al. Combined genetic profiles of components and reg-ulators of the vitamin K-dependent gamma-carboxylation system affect individual sensitiv-ity to warfarin. Thromb Haemost 2006;95(2):205–11.

[40] Chen LY, Eriksson N, Gwilliam R, et al. Gamma-glutamyl carboxylase (GGCX) microsa-tellite and warfarin dosing. Blood 2005;106(10):3673–4.

[41] Darghouth D, Hallgren KW, Shtofman RL, et al. Compound heterozygosity of novel mis-sense mutations in the gamma-glutamyl-carboxylase gene causes hereditary combined vita-min K-dependent coagulation factor deficiency. Blood 2006;108(6):1925–31.

[42] Hylek EM, Evans-Molina C, Shea C, et al. Major hemorrhage and tolerability of warfarin in the first year of therapy among elderly patients with atrial fibrillation. Circulation 2007; 115(21):2689–96.

[43] Ma JD, Nafziger AN, Kashuba AD, et al. Limited sampling strategy of S-warfarin concen-trations, but not warfarin S/R ratios, accurately predicts S-warfarin AUC during baseline and inhibition in CYP2C9 extensive metabolizers. J Clin Pharmacol 2004;44(6):570–6.

[44] Check W. Too fast or too slow on PGx testing? CAP Today, March 2008. Available at: http:// www.cap.org/apps/cap.portal?_nfpb = true&cntvwrPtlt_actionOverride = %2Fportlets% 2FcontentViewer%2Fshow&_windowLabel = cntvwrPtlt&cntvwrPtlt%7BactionForm. contentReference%7D = cap_today%2Fcover_stories%2F0308_TooFastOrSlow.html&_ state = maximized&_pageLabel = cntv. Accessed May 2, 2008.

[45] Bussey HI, Wittkowsky AK, Hylek EM, et al. Genetic testing for warfarin dosing? Not yet ready for prime time. Pharmacotherapy 2008;28(2):141–3.

[46] Warfarin dosing. Available at: www.warfarindosing.org. Accessed May 2, 2008.

[47] Valdes R, Jr. Computational decision-making supprot tool for incorporating PGx-testing to Warfarin therapeudics. Presented at Molecular Medicine. Applying current and emerging technologies. Lake Buena, FL; March 29, 2008.

[48] Hylek EM, D'Antonio J, Evans-Molina C, et al. Translating the results of randomized trials into clinical practice: the challenge of warfarin candidacy among hospitalized elderly patients with atrial fibrillation. Stroke 2006;37(4):1075–80.

[49] Garcia DA, Regan S, Crowther M, et al. The risk of hemorrhage among patients with warfarin-associated coagulopathy. J Am Coll Cardiol 2006;47(4):804–8.

[50] Higashi MK, Veenstra DL, Kondo LM, et al. Association between CYP2C9 genetic variants and anticoagulation-related outcomes during warfarin therapy. JAMA 2002;287(13): 1690–8.

[51] Hill CE, Duncan A, Wirth D, et al. Detection and identification of cytochrome P-450 2C9 alleles *1, *2, and *3 by high-resolution melting curve analysis of PCR amplicons. Am J Clin Pathol 2006;125(4):584–91.

[52] Hillman MA, Wilke RA, Yale SH, et al. A prospective, randomized pilot trial of model-based warfarin dose initiation using CYP2C9 genotype and clinical data. Clin Med Res 2005;3(3):137–45.

[53] Wen MS, Lee M, Chen JJ, et al. Prospective study of warfarin dosage requirements based on CYP2C9 and VKORC1 genotypes. Clin Pharmacol Ther 2008;84(1):83–9.

[54] Baudhuin LM, Langman LJ, O'Kane DJ. Translation of pharmacogenetics into clinically relevant testing modalities. Clin Pharmacol Ther 2007;82(4):373–6.

[55] Flockhart DA, O'Kane D, Williams MS, et al. Pharmacogenetic testing of CYP2C9 and VKORC1 alleles for warfarin. Genet Med 2008;10(2):139–50.

[56] Gage BF, Lesko LJ. Pharmacogenetics of warfarin: regulatory, scientific, and clinical issues. J Thromb Thrombolysis 2008;25(1):45–51.

[57] Linder MW, Looney S, Adams JE 3rd, et al. Warfarin dose adjustments based on CYP2C9 genetic polymorphisms. J Thromb Thrombolysis 2002;14(3):227–32.

[58] Grice GR, Milligan PE, Eby C, et al. Pharmacogenetic dose refinement prevents warfarin overdose in a patient who is highly warfarin-sensitive. Thromb Haemost 2008;6(1):207–9.

[59] McWilliam A, Lutter R, Nardinelli C. Health care savings from personalized medicine using genetic testing: the case for warfarin. AEI- Brookings Joint Center for Regulatory Studies, 2006. Available at: http://aei-brookings.org/publications/abstract.php?pid = 1127. Accessed March 20, 2008.

ELSEVIER
SAUNDERS

CLINICS IN
LABORATORY
MEDICINE

Clin Lab Med 28 (2008) 525–537

Pharmacogenetic Testing for Warfarin Sensitivity

Elaine Lyon, PhD[a,b,*], Gwen McMillin, PhD[a,b],
Roberta Melis, PhD[b]

[a]Department of Pathology, University of Utah, Salt Lake City, Utah, USA
[b]ARUP Institute for Clinical and Experimental Pathology, Salt Lake City, Utah, USA

The goal of pharmacogenetic testing is to predict the right drug at the right dose for each patient by incorporating a patient's genetic profile in drug and dose selection decisions. This goal appears achievable in dosing for warfarin, with the hope of decreasing the incidence and severity of adverse events, particularly bleeding episodes. By using knowledge of the metabolic and the signaling pathways and gene variants affecting warfarin metabolism, a mathematical model to predict initial or maintenance dose is possible.

The US Food and Drug Administration (FDA) recently mandated that genotyping information be included in the warfarin product label as a possible companion test for prescribing warfarin. The information is specific for warfarin sensitivity because of well-characterized variants of the CYP2C9 gene and a promoter variant in the VKORC1 gene. The cytochrome p450 isozyme 2C9 is the primary enzyme involved with inactivating s-warfarin. CYP2C9 genetic variants decrease enzyme activity and impair metabolism, slowing clearance and causing an accumulation of s-warfarin. Thus, lower warfarin doses are associated with CYP2C9 variants. Common variants in 2C9 in Caucasians are *2 (c.430C>T; p.R144C) and *3 (c.1075A>C; p.I259L). Although both decrease activity, two copies of *2 do so by 30% to 40%, while two copies of *3 decrease activity over 50% [1]. The enzyme vitamin K epoxide reductase (VKOR) is important to vitamin K recycling and is the primary target for warfarin. Thus, inhibition of VKOR represents the pharmacodynamics of warfarin. A common promoter variant in VKORC1, the gene complex that encodes

---

* Corresponding author. ARUP Laboratories, 500 Chipeta Way, Salt Lake City, UT 84108.
E-mail address: lyone@aruplab.com (E. Lyon).

0272-2712/08/$ - see front matter © 2008 Elsevier Inc. All rights reserved.
doi:10.1016/j.cll.2008.09.001 *labmed.theclinics.com*

for VKOR (VKORC1 c.−1639G>A), alters the expression of the receptor, resulting in decreased concentrations of VKOR [2]. Variants of VKORC1 and CYP2C9 may explain up to 50% of the interindividual variability to warfarin [1]. Due, in part, of the recent inclusion of genetic information (CYP2C9 and VKORC1) in the warfarin labeling, laboratories are offering warfarin testing; manufacturers are developing warfarin sensitivity assays; and the College of American Pathologists (CAP) is offering proficiency testing.

This article describes testing technologies available for warfarin sensitivity testing, including laboratory-developed assays and reagents from manufacturers that are currently available commercially. Hybridization probes (Idaho Technology, Salt Lake City, Utah), signal amplification (Third Wave Technologies, Madison, Wisconsin), and microarrays including bead arrays (Luminex; Molecular Diagnostics, Toronto, Canada) and solid-surface arrays (Osmetech and Autogenomics, Passadena, California) are discussed. A summary of the variants detected with each method is shown in Table 1. The technologies are discussed without regard to DNA extraction techniques. Laboratory testing issues, however, including acceptable sample types and potential assay limitations, turn-around time, and quality controls are discussed.

Hybridization probes

Hybridization probes are used routinely to test small panels of mutations, and are well suited for this application. In principle, this combines real-time polymerase chain reaction (PCR) followed by a slow melt analysis. Probes covering a mutation of interest are included with PCR. Hybridization assays first were described using fluorescent resonance energy transfer (FRET). The most commonly used chemistry is dual adjacent hybridization probes, each labeled with a single fluorophore. One probe is designed to hybridize to the region of the mutation or variant and is referred to as the mutation probe or detection probe. The other is designed with a higher melting temperature (Tm) and is referred to as the anchor probe [3]. In the LightCycler system, where this first was described, the fluorophores are often fluorescein and LCRed 640 or 705. As the template is amplified, probes hybridize, and the fluorophores are brought into close proximity. The donor fluorophore transmits its energy to the acceptor fluorophore of the adjacent probe. This fluorophore then emits its energy at a longer wavelength, which is detected by the instrument. Upon denaturation, the probes dissociate at a specific Tm, resulting in a loss of fluorescence. A mismatch between the probe and its template lowers the Tm. Results are displayed as derivative of fluorescence and temperature (dF/dT).

Another hybridization probe design includes a single fluorescently labeled probe [4]. In this case, fluorescence is transferred by a G on the opposite strand, but adjacent to the labeled end of the probe. Fluorescence is

Table 1
Variants in warfarin sensitivity testing methods

Gene variants	Nucleotide position	Nucleotide change	Amino acid	Gene region	ITI simple probes	Invader	xTAG	INFINITI	eSensor[b]
CYP2C9									
*2	c.430	C>T	p.R144C	Exon 3	■	■	■	■	■
*3	c.1075	A>C	p.L359I	Exon 7	■	■	■	■	■
*4	c.1076	T>C	p.I359T	Exon 7			■	■	
*5	c.1080	C>G	p.D360E	Exon 5			■	■	■
*6	c.818	delA	p.273 FS*	Exon 7				■	■
*11	c.1003	C>T	p.R335W	Exon 7				■	■
*14	c.374	G>A	p.R125H	Exon 3				■	■
*15	c.485	C>A	p.S162X	Exon 4				■	■
*16	c.895	A>G	p.T299A	Exon 6				■	■
VKORC1									
3673	c.−1639	G>A		Promoter				■	
5808	c.173+324	T>G		Intron 1				■	
6009	c.173+525	C>T		Intron 1				■	
6484	c.173+1000	C>T		Intron 1				■	
6853	c.283+124	G>C		Intron 2				■	
7566	c.283+837+C>T	C>T		Intron 2				■	
8773	c.538	C>T	p.L120L	Exon 3	■	■	■	■	
9041	c.492+134	G>A		3′-UTR					
85	g.85	G>T	p.V29L	Exon 1			■		
121	g.121	G>T	p.A41S	Exon 1			■		
134	g.134	T>C	p.V45A	Exon 1			■		
172	g.172	A>G	p.V66M	Exon 1			■		
1331	g.1331	G>A	p.L128R	Exon 2			■		
3487	g.3487	T>G		Exon 3			■		
CYP4F2									
	g.1347	G>A	p.V433M	Exon 11					■

Abbreviation: FS, frame shift.
[b] IVD product includes only CYP2C9 *2,*3 and VKORC1 -1639.

quenched, and released upon denaturation. The ease of designing hybridiza-tion probes makes this technology suitable for a laboratory-developed test.

Hybridization probe reagents for warfarin are commercially available from Idaho Technology, Inc (ITI Simpleprobe). The chemistry is based on a single fluorescent probe. Three separate (nonmultiplexed) reactions are performed, using the same conditions. The authors typically use 50 ng of DNA for clinical testing, although much less may be required. The deriv-ative melting curves are displayed separately for each mutation (Fig. 1). The throughput allows eight samples, each with three reactions, plus six controls per run on the LightCycler, which holds 32 samples. To increase through-put, other instruments such as the LC480 (Roche Molecular Systems, Indi-anapolis, Indiana) or the LightScanner (Idaho Technology) allow the same chemistry in a 96 or 384 sample format. PCR and detection can be per-formed in less than 1 hour, making it suitable for rapid turnaround. The probes are all perfect matches to the targeted mutation (CYP2C9 *2, *3 and VKORC1 -1689G > A). By designing probes to match the mutation, the possibility of false positives from other mutations that may be within the region of the probe is reduced. For example, if a mutation other than the target mutation is on the opposite chromosome from the targeted muta-tion, the probe would have two mismatches with the template (one with the wild-type base at the targeted mutation position and one additional), which would destabilize the probe further and result in a lower Tm than the wild-type Tm. In an earlier version of these reagents, a rare variant caused a false-positive result, because the probe was a perfect match to the wild type. Additionally, the Tms of the target mutation and rare mu-tation with one mismatch could not be distinguished [5]. Because of this, the probes were redesigned to match the mutation. This technology has been used for several warfarin studies [5,6].

A similar technology relies on hydrolysis probes, namely, Taqman chem-istry. Two probes are designed, one a perfect match to the normal allele and one to the mutant or variant allele. In Taqman chemistry, probes are re-leased from quenching when the Taq polymerase degrades the probe, releas-ing the fluorophore into solution. This technology was developed from Applied Biosystems (Foster City, California) and is compatible with the 7900 real-time instrument (Applied Biosystems). Taqman chemistry also is developed easily by individual laboratories [7].

Invader

A signal amplification method (Invader chemistry, Third Wave Technol-ogies) for the three most common genetic variants associated with warfarin sensitivity is available through Third Wave Technologies. This method in-volves a multiplex PCR reaction designed to amplify regions important to detecting the two most common alleles of CYP2C9 (*2, *3), and VKORC1 −1639G > A using a standard thermal cycler and primers provided by Third

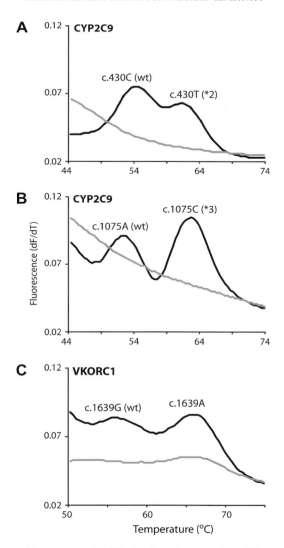

Fig. 1. Derivative melting curves using ITI simple probes, showing wild-type (wt) and variant alleles. Heterozygous, no template control. In each case, the probe is a perfect match to the variant allele. Heterozygous (black line), no template control (grey line).

Wave [8]. Approximately 50 to 150 ng of DNA is required. Following amplification, two simultaneous Invader reactions (isothermal) are performed per variant. Specifically, a three-stranded structure is formed through hybridization of two Invader probes to complimentary regions of the target DNA. The three-stranded structure is comprised of the target DNA and two probes, one of which overlaps by one base with the other two, thus creating a flap on the 5' end that does not hybridize. A proprietary cleavase recognizes the overlapping structure and releases the flap plus one nucleotide. The probes rapidly cycle on and off of the target DNA so that multiple probe molecules are cleaved, generating many flaps per target DNA during this part of the reaction. In a secondary Invader reaction, flaps hybridize to complimentary FRET probes. Cleavage of the FRET probe releases the fluorophore from the quencher, generating a unique fluorescent signal. The signal is amplified because of generation of many flaps per target DNA and the cleavage of many flaps from the FRET probes [9]. It is estimated that 1–10 million cleavage products are generated per target sequence. Fluorescence is measured using a fluorescence plate reader such as the Tecan GENios fluorometer (Tecan Systems, Durham, North Carolina). The process requires approximately 3 hours after DNA extraction. Genotypes are called based on allelic ratios and thresholds established by Third Wave.

The Invader method is attractive to a laboratory with little genetic testing experience, because it is easy to perform, relatively fast, and requires little investment in equipment. Because only the three most common variants associated with warfarin sensitivity are included, the failure rate for the assay is low (less than 10% in the authors' hands), and results are also relatively easy to interpret. This method, one of the first commercially available, is used by most laboratories that participated in the CAP proficiency testing survey for pharmacogenetics testing in 2007 [10]. The throughput for this assay is designed for the 96-well plate format. In the current reagent system, 28 samples (three reactions for each) can be genotyped on a single 96-well plate. The technology also is used for various infectious disease and molecular genetic testing applications.

Microarrays

Microarray technologies allow for detection of multiple variants and polymorphisms within a single test. Most microarray technologies involve some form of multiplexed allele-specific DNA amplification, hybridization to a solid surface, and either optical or electronic detection methods. The following are descriptions of three microarray platforms that have been applied to warfarin pharmacogenetics: the xTAG bead array (Luminex Molecular Diagnostics Corporation) and the INFINITI BioFilmChip array (Autogenomics, Inc., Carlsbad, California) that both use fluorescence detection, and the eSensor gold electrode array (Osmetech Molecular Diagnostics Toronto, Canada) that uses electrochemical detection.

xTAG CYP2C9-VKORC1 assay

The xTAG P450-2C9 + VKORC1 assay (Luminex Molecular Diagnostics) is based on xTAG technology [11], a universal color-coded bead array operating on the Luminex xMAP IS System (Luminex Corporation). Each bead is characterized by a unique signature, determined by a mixture of red and infrared fluorophores and a universal antitag sequence. The detection of fluorescent signals is performed using the Luminex analyzer, with two lasers that identify each microsphere particle, and capture the fluorescence of the reporter dye. Briefly, a primary multiplex PCR of the CYP2C9 and VKORC1 gene regions, including 12 allelic variants [8,12] is performed with 25 to 50 ng DNA and followed by a shrimp alkaline phosphatase and exonuclease I (EXO/SAP) cleanup step, to enable efficient incorporation of biotin-dCTP during the allele-specific primer extension (ASPE) reaction. Each allele-specific primer is characterized at the 5' end by a unique 24-oligomer DNA tag, while the 3' sequence of the primer is specific to the allele. In the ASPE reaction, primers for both the mutant and wild-type forms of each variant are included. During the ASPE reaction, a thermophilic DNA polymerase extends and incorporates biotin dCTP only when the correct primer hybridizes the allele sequence. A noncomplementary primer will not be extended or labeled because of the 3' mismatch base. During the hybridization step, the ASPE products are hybridized to complementary oligonucleotide sequences (antitag) that are affixed to specific Luminex beads. The beads then are incubated in a fluorescent reporter solution (Strepavidin-R-phycoerythrin conjugate), and fluorescence intensities are measured by the Luminex xMAP system [13]. Genotype calls are determined by the Tag-It data analysis software (TDAS) (Luminex Molecular Diagnostics). With a 96-well format, 90 to 94 samples can be performed at once with two to six controls. Collecting data from the plate reader is rapid (approximately 10 minutes), so multiple plates may be read if a higher throughput is desired.

INFINITI 2C9-VKORC1 assay

This assay is based on a BioFilmChip Microarray, a film-based matrix for the retention of an oligonucleotide array, on the INFINITI Analyzer system (Autogenomics, Incorporated), and is cleared as an in vitro diagnostic (IVD). The INFINITI Analyzer is an automated, multiplexing, continuous flow microarray platform that integrates the discrete test processes for the analysis of DNA, such as sample handling, reagent management, hybridization, stringency, and detection, into a totally self-contained system. The INFINITI Analyzer features include: a temperature cycler for denaturing nucleic acids and performing allele-specific primer extension, a thermal hybridization incubator, and an optics system comprised of a built-in confocal microscope with two lasers. A primary multiplex PCR of the CYP2C9 and VKORC1 gene regions, including 14 allelic variants, is performed and then loaded onto the INFINITI Analyzer. The following steps are automated and performed by the INFINITI Analyzer:

Detection primer extension (DPE); in this step, allele-specific primers, tailed with a unique antizip code sequence, are extended, and fluorescently labeled dCTPs are incorporated by DNA polymerase carried over from the first PCR

DNA hybridization of the DPE products to the corresponding zip code oligonucleotides spotted on the BioFilmChip

A washing step to remove the unbound primers

Fluorescence signal acquisition, on BioFilmChip, by optical module

Fluorescent signal intensities are analyzed by INFINITI Qmatic software and correlated to genotype-based on allelic ratios and manufacturer established cut-off thresholds

PCR multiplexing and post-PCR automation make this platform attractive to laboratories. The throughput is less scalable than the previous platforms described, but can process up to 22 samples plus two controls. The starting PCR uses approximately 50 ng of DNA. After PCR, the automated platform takes 4 hours until the first results, with 30 minutes for each subsequent sample.

eSensor

The eSensor microarray is based on a printed circuit board containing gold electrodes for detection of specific nucleic acids in a sandwich-based assay design [14,15]. The hybridization and detection components of the assay are performed within a microfluidic cartridge, using automated instrumentation (XT-8) (Osmetech Molecular Diagnostics). Ten SNPs are targeted: eight SNPs in CYP2C9 for detection of *2, *3, *5, *6, *11, *14, *15, and *16 alleles (Table 1), -1639G>A in VKORC1, and V433M in CYP4F2 [16]. Results for all but the *CYP2C9* *2, *3, and VKORC1 -1639G>A genotypes, however, are masked by software in the in vitro diagnostic. This assay, which includes detection of just the three well-characterized variants, has received clearance from the FDA. Accuracy of the method has been established through 100% agreement of eSensor genotype results with bidirectional DNA sequencing. The assay reagents include a complete PCR reagent containing primers and dNTPs, DNA polymerase, exonuclease, signal probes, buffers, and cartridges (in packages of eight). The assay is designed to be performed in groups of up to eight samples, wherein one sample (patient, control, or otherwise) is analyzed per cartridge. Cartridges have stability of approximately 1 week at room temperature once the package of eight has been opened. The XT-8 instrument is designed so that each cartridge slot is independent; therefore the instrument could function in a random access mode. The assay can be performed within 4 hours after DNA extraction.

The assay begins with DNA (10 to 1000 ng) that is amplified by multiplexed PCR using a standard thermal cycler, followed by a bacteriophage λ exonuclease digestion to remove the nontarget amplicon strands. A mixture of amplicon, signal probes, and buffer is loaded into a cartridge, and the cartridges loaded into an XT-8 instrument. The instrument is modular in design, to accommodate one to three towers that each contain eight cartridge slots, so that larger groups of samples can be accommodated. The instrument interface allows users to determine the sample identity, initiate assay protocols, view assay progress, and analyze the data. Once the assay protocol is initiated on the XT-8, a hybridization protocol allows the target DNA to hybridize to complementary capture probes that are immobilized to gold electrodes in the cartridge; the capture probe for each SNP is localized on a different electrode. Each capture probe is designed to bind both the wild-type and variant SNP of a given allele. The signal probes hybridize to a second region of the target DNA containing the SNP sequence, forming a three-complex structure. The signal probes are allele-specific, and incorporate electrochemically active ferrocene labels to distinguish wild-type and variant sequences. When hybridized to the target DNA, these labels become physically located in close proximity to the gold electrodes to allow detection and genotyping. The ferrous ion within each ferrocene group undergoes cyclic oxidation and reduction, leading to loss or gain of electrons. The resulting current is measured using alternating current voltammetry, and harmonic signal analysis is used to discriminate the ferrocene-dependent faradic current from background capacitive current. The gold electrodes are coated with oligonucleotide capture probes within an insulating self-assembled monolayer [17]. Genotypes are called by the ratio of signals generated by the pairs of ferrocene labels, which are specific for each allele, and the manufacturer establishes thresholds.

Single nucleotide primer extension

A multiplexed technology that is simple to design and perform is a single nucleotide extension assay (SNE). The chemistry is based on the di-deoxy single nucleotide extension of an unlabelled oligonucleotide primer. Typically up to 12 variants may be detected in a reaction. Either a multiplexed PCR or long-range PCR is used as a first step. This is followed by a multiplexed reaction containing SNE primers and SNapShot reagents (Applied Bioscience, Foster City, California), including AmpliTaq DNA polymerase and fluorescently labeled di-deoxy nucleotides (ddNTPs). Each SNE primer is designed one nucleotide away from the mutation of interest and with a difference of four to six nucleotides between primer lengths, allowing size separation electrophoretically. The polymerase extends the primer by one nucleotide, adding a single fluorescently labeled ddNTP. The resulting reactions are separated by capillary electrophoresis. The combination of color and size identifies each position and the base that is added (complementary to the mutation or wild-type). Although this technology has not been described for a warfarin assay, it is well suited for a laboratory-developed test [18] for warfarin sensitivity.

Pyrosequencing

Pyrosequencing also has been described in testing these variants [8,19]. This technology is used to sequence small stretches of DNA and is well-suited for warfarin sensitivity testing in a laboratory with this sequencing expertise. Essentially the pyrosequencing method allows sequencing of a single-strand DNA (ssDNA) by synthesizing the complementary strand along it, one base pair at a time, and detecting which base has been added. Sequencing primers are designed to be within a few bases of the targeted mutation, and hybridize to the ssDNA in presence of the enzymes DNA polymerase, ATP sulfurylase, luciferase, and apyrase and substrates adenosine 5'phosphate and luciferin. Light is produced only when the correct complementary nucleotide bases are incorporated onto the template. This incorporation releases pyrophosphate (PPi) stoichiometrically. The adenosine triphosphate (ATP) sulfurylase quantitatively converts PPi to ATP, which in turn acts as an energy donor of the luciferase-mediated conversion of luciferin to oxyluciferin. This generates visible light in amounts that are proportional to the amount of ATP and relative to the number of each nucleotide incorporated. Unincorporated nucleotides and ATP are degraded by the apyrase, and the reaction begins again with another nucleotide.

Implementing warfarin sensitivity testing

Implementing this testing in the laboratory poses several challenges. Laboratories choose technologies based on existing instrumentation and expertise in the laboratory, and the mutations for their testing population. Studies have focused on Caucasian populations; however, other ethnic groups also display warfarin sensitivity. The maximum number of mutations detected by the platforms described here is 14. Other mutations within these genes also may contribute to warfarin sensitivity. Additional genes that contribute to the inheritability of warfarin sensitivity or warfarin resistance include protein C, microsomal epoxide hydrolase-1, gamma-glutamyl carboxylase, orosomucoid 2, calumenin, and apolipoprotein E [20–23]; however, their contribution may be minor compared with additional environmental or clinical factors. In general, genes and variants associated with warfarin resistance are not included in studies focused on warfarin genotyping.

Turn-around times may be important in choosing a platform for different clinical indications. Emergency situations will require testing to be performed in hospital laboratories to obtain results within a few hours. This need, however, essentially is based on logistics and operational control rather than clinical need, because efficacy of warfarin requires washout of existing vitamin K- dependent clotting factors, which may require a few days. In most circumstances, having results within 3 to 5 days after initiation of warfarin (before the first dose adjustment) may be sufficient. In cases of planned surgery, testing can be performed and results received as part of a presurgery workup.

The starting analyte for all these assays is purified DNA. Pharmacogenetic testing lends itself well to DNA extracted from blood, saliva, or buccal swabs. Decisions about acceptable sample type should be based on the required DNA input for the method and the sample types cleared by the FDA.

Ensuring ongoing accuracy of an assay is a requirement for all Clinical Laboratory Improvement Act (CLIA) certified laboratories as part of a laboratory's quality assurance program. One way to comply with this requirement is through proficiency testing. An external proficiency testing program for warfarin sensitivity is offered through CAP. In a 2007 survey, 18 laboratories participated. The analytic agreement was excellent by all methods of testing [10].

Effectively communicating results to physicians is a critical component of laboratory testing. The reports should list the mutations detected, because this will vary among laboratories. Standard nomenclature has been recommended, but may be confusing as literature reports different nomenclature. For example, in the literature, VKORC1 results may refer to haplotype A groups (low dose) or haplotype B groups (high dose). Haplotype A group (haplotype 1 and 2) includes the -1639A allele, while B (haplotype 7, 8, and 9) corresponds to the -1639G allele [24]. A variant in linkage disequilibrium with $-1639G>A$ variant is the intronic variant $1173C>T$, and some reagents or laboratories may choose to test this variant instead of the promoter variant [24,25]. For CYP2C9, standard nomenclatures for the nucleic acids and proteins are $c.430C>T$ and $c.1075A>C$, and p.R144C and p.I259L, respectively. The common nomenclature in most literature is by allele nomenclature, such as *2 and *3. Familiar nomenclature often is preferred over standard, and potentially both may be used in the report.

Whether the laboratory should give dosing recommendations is controversial. To do so, laboratories need to collect more information than typically is provided, such as height, weight, clinical status (eg, diagnosis and liver function), and concomitant medications. In providing these recommendations, laboratories may be involved in the practice of medicine to a greater extent than they have been in the past, without having a direct relationship with the patient. As dosing algorithms are refined, however, laboratories may be able to guide physicians in treatment.

Challenges exist in incorporating genotyping as standard of care. Despite the FDA-required warfarin label update, adoption of sensitivity genotyping by physicians has been limited; however, growth of use is increasing. Establishing the utility of warfarin sensitivity genotyping is essential in realizing its potential in preventing bleeding episodes. Questions remain as to its use in establishing starting or maintenance doses, and how to incorporate genotyping into patient management.

References

[1] Sconce EA, Khan TI, Wynne HA, et al. The impact of CYP2C9 and VKORC1 genetic polymorphism and patient characteristics upon warfarin dose requirements: proposal for a new dosing regimen. Blood 2005;106:2329–33.

[2] Wang D, Chen H, Momary KM, et al. Regulatory polymorphism in vitamin K epoxide reductase complex subunit 1 (VKORC1) affects gene expression and warfarin dose requirement. Blood 2008;112:1013–21.

[3] Bernard PS, Ajioka RS, Kushner JP, et al. Homogeneous multiplex genotyping of hemochromatosis mutations with fluorescent hybridization probes. Am J Pathol 1998;153: 1055–61.

[4] Crockett AO, Wittwer CT. Fluorescein-labeled oligonucleotides for real-time PCR: using the inherent quenching of deoxyguanosine nucleotides. Anal Biochem 2001;290:89–97.

[5] Carlquist JF, McKinney JT, Nicholas ZP, et al. Rapid melting curve analysis for genetic variants that underlie interindividual variability in stable warfarin dosing. J Thromb Thrombolysis 2008;26:1–7.

[6] Haug KB, Sharikabad MN, Kringen NK, et al. Warfarin dose and INR related to genotypes of CYP2C9 and VKORC1 in patients with myocardial infarction. Thromb J 2008;6:7.

[7] Carlquist JF, Horne BD, Muhlestein JB, et al. Genotypes of the cytochrome p450 isoform, CYP2C9, and the vitamin K epoxide reductase complex subunit 1 conjointly determine stable warfarin dose: a prospective study. J Thromb Thrombolysis 2006;22:191–7.

[8] King CR, Porche-Sorbet RM, Gage BF, et al. Performance of commercial platforms for rapid genotyping of polymorphisms affecting warfarin dose. Am J Clin Pathol 2008;129: 876–83.

[9] Third Wave Technologies. Invader. Avaliable at: http://www.twt.com/invader/invader. html. Accessed July 28, 2008.

[10] Participant summary report: PGX-B. The CAP Pharmacogenetics Working Group, CAP/ ACMG Molecular Genetics Committee 2007, 6–8.

[11] Zhu Y, Shennan M, Reynolds KK, et al. Estimation of warfarin maintenance dose based on VKORC1 (-1639 G $>$ A) and CYP2C9 genotypes. Clin Chem 2007;53:1199–205.

[12] Scott SA, Edelmann L, Kornreich R, et al. Warfarin pharmacogenetics: CYP2C9 and VKORC1 genotypes predict different sensitivity and resistance frequencies in the Ashkenazi and Sephardi Jewish populations. Am J Hum Genet 2008;82:495–500.

[13] Luminex. What is xTAG technology. Avaliable at: http://www.luminexcorp.com/ technology/xtag/index.html. Accessed July 27, 2008.

[14] Umek RM, Lin SW, Vielmetter J, et al. Electronic detection of nucleic acids: a versatile platform for molecular diagnostics. J Mol Diagn 2001;3:74–84.

[15] Reed MR, Coty WA. eSensor: a microarray technology based on electrochemical detection of nucleic acids and its application to cystic fibrosis carrier screening, in microarrays: preparation, detection methods, data analysis, and applications. In: Dill K, Liu R, Grodzinski P, editors. Kluwer: Springer-Verlag; 2008; in press.

[16] Caldwell MD, Awad T, Johnson JA, et al. CYP4F2 genetic variant alters required warfarin dose. Blood 2008;111:4106–12.

[17] Coty B, Reed M, Jacobs A, et al. Development and evaluation of an eSensor genotyping test for CYP450 2C9 and VKORC1 polymorphisms Avaliable at: http://www.osmetech.com/ pdf/PosterAMP11-07.pdf. Accessed July 27, 2008.

[18] Jama M, Nelson L, Pont-Kingdon G, et al. Simultaneous amplification, detection, and analysis of common mutations in the galactose-1-phosphate uridyl transferase gene. J Mol Diagn 2007;9:618–23.

[19] Enstrom C, Osman A, Lindahl TL. A genotyping method for VKORC1 1173C $>$ T by Pyrosequencing technology. Scand J Clin Lab Invest 2007;21:1–4.

[20] Krynetskiy E, McDonnell P. Building individualized medicine: prevention of adverse reactions to warfarin therapy. J Pharmacol Exp Ther 2007;322:427–34.

[21] Shikata E, Ieiri I, Ishiguro S, et al. Association of pharmacokinetic (CYP2C9) and pharmacodynamic (factors II, VII, IX, and X; proteins S and C; and gamma-glutamyl carboxylase) gene variants with warfarin sensitivity. Blood 2004;103:2630–5.

[22] Kimmel SE, Christie J, Kealey C, et al. Apolipoprotein E genotype and warfarin dosing among Caucasians and African Americans. Pharmacogenomics J 2008;8:53–60.

[23] Vecsler M, Loebstein R, Almog S, et al. Combined genetic profiles of components and regulators of the vitamin K-dependent gamma-carboxylation system affect individual sensitivity to warfarin. Thromb Haemost 2006;95:205–11.

[24] Rieder MJ, Reiner AP, Gage BF, et al. Effect of VKORC1 haplotypes on transcriptional regulation and warfarin dose. N Engl J Med 2005;352:2285–93.

[25] Kosaki K, Yamaghishi C, Sato R, et al. 1173C>T polymorphism in VKORC1 modulates the required warfarin dose. Pediatr Cardiol 2006;27(6):685–8.

CLINICS IN
LABORATORY
MEDICINE

Clin Lab Med 28 (2008) 539–552

Dynamic Pharmacogenetic Models in Anticoagulation Therapy

Marjorie Bon Homme, PhD[a],
Kristen K. Reynolds, PhD[a,b],
Roland Valdes, Jr, PhD, FACB[a],
Mark W. Linder, PhD[a,*]

[a]Department of Pathology and Laboratory Medicine, University of Louisville,
501 South Floyd Street, MDR-218, Louisville, KY 40202, USA
[b]PGXL Laboratories, 201 East Jefferson Street, Suite 309, Louisville, KY 40202, USA

How may a combination of biophysical techniques (single nucleotide polymorphism detection) and bioinformatics (pharmacologic principles) be combined to provide information suitable for medical intervention? Sequencing of the human genome was made possible by combining the application of tools involving sophisticated biophysical techniques and advanced bioinformatics. Converting known changes in genetic structure into meaningful diagnostic information poses significant challenges and begs the question of how might the medical community leverage this knowledge to provide a more "personalized" medicine approach to therapeutics. Typically, physiologic models are routinely used to teach theory and mechanisms to medical students, residents, and interns. When the applications involve higher-level mathematics or integration of numerous patient cofactors, these complex physiologic models must be reduced to simple algorithms. The paradigm is now shifting toward managing patients based on genetic information unique for that individual and with the aid of computational decision-support tools. The purpose of this article is to demonstrate how a dynamic clinical-support tool can guide individualized drug therapy. We use the drug warfarin as a model to demonstrate how pharmacogenetics when combined with fundamental principles of pharmacokinetic and pharmacodynamics can provide a powerful decision-support tool to optimize personalized therapeutics.

This work was supported by Grant No. K23AA014235ML and R44 HL 090055KR.

* Corresponding author. Department of Pathology and Laboratory Medicine, University of Louisville, 511 South Floyd Street, MDR-218, Louisville, KY 40202.

E-mail address: mwlind01@louisville.edu (M.W. Linder).

doi:10.1016/j.cll.2008.10.002
labmed.theclinics.com

Warfarin, the most commonly prescribed oral anticoagulant [1], is also one of the top two drugs implicated in serious adverse events by The Adverse Event Reporting System (AERS) of the US Food and Drug Administration [1,2]. Warfarin owes its membership in the AERS database to its narrow therapeutic index (INR between 2.0 and 3.0) and high interindividual variability in maintenance dose requirement (0.5 to 60 mg/d). A "standard dose" can cause life-threatening hemorrhage or fail to prevent a stroke. Avoiding these adverse drug reactions could potentially save the health care system anywhere from $100 million to $2 billion [3] annually in addition to the incalculable increase in quality of life and decreased morbidity.

The difficulties in managing patients on warfarin have fueled the interest in identification of sources of variability in response and for methods for reducing this variability. These efforts have led to the discovery of inherited genetic polymorphisms that alter the pharmacokinetics and pharmacodynamics of warfarin such that a compensatory dosage modification is required to optimize therapy. It is now well established that inherited differences in the gene encoding the cytochrome P4502C9 (CYP2C9) lead to decreased S-warfarin clearance and therefore require a compensatory dosage reduction to yield the appropriate therapeutic concentration under steady-state conditions. Further, it is now well accepted that inherited differences in the expression of the gene encoding the vitamin K epoxide reductase complex subunit 1 (VKORC1) have an effect on the pharmacodynamics of warfarin. Our group has evidence that the basis for this effect is related to the threshold concentrations of S-warfarin required to sufficiently inhibit the activity of this complex to result in a therapeutic increase in the prothrombin time [4]. Since the discovery of these inherited differences, this field has witnessed an evolution in the tools that apply this knowledge. The earliest applications involved retrospective grouping of patients by their genetic category and using the mean maintenance dose for that genetic category to make prospective predictions. This categorical approach was then replaced by multivariate mathematical equations that include clinical features of the patient, in addition to the CYP2C9 and VKORC1 genotypes, leading to higher resolution tools for estimating warfarin dose. The next step in this evolution of application is to build methods that increase the ability to apply this information in an ongoing manner, taking into account the individual's dosing history and INR response. To achieve this level of application requires a transition from statistical association to mechanism-based application. One approach for capturing the mechanism-based effects of these genetic variants is through the application of a dynamic clinical decision support tool. Our view of the features and benefits of such a tool are listed in Box 1.

VKORC1 genotype and warfarin dose requirement

Warfarin is a racemic mixture of R- and S-enantiomers and exerts its antithrombotic effect by inhibiting its target enzyme vitamin K epoxide

---

Box 1. Benefits of dynamic modeling for safe and effective anticoagulation therapy

Features
- Must be based on validated components.
- Empower practitioner with information needed to guide their judgment.
- Application where simultaneous and conflicting variables must be reconciled.
- Yield more information than the sum of the individual inputs.

Benefits
- Manage the increasing complexity of clinical laboratory data.
- Reconcile interdependency between laboratory, clinical and other diagnostic information.
- Enable sustained application of diagnostic information.
- New opportunities for reporting of laboratory data as information.

---

reductase (VKOR). S-warfarin is three to five times more potent at inhibiting VKOR than R-warfarin and is therefore considered to be the active form. Inhibiting VKOR decreases the pool of reduced vitamin K necessary to activate enzymes involved in the coagulation pathway, namely factors II, VII, IX, and X, and proteins C, S, and Z. VKOR is encoded by VKOR complex subunit 1 gene (VKORC1).

Differences in VKORC1 expression, as a result of genetic polymorphisms, are responsible for about 15% to 30% of warfarin dose variability [5–9]. In 2005, numerous studies reported evidence of an association between VKORC1 polymorphisms and warfarin sensitivity or low dose requirement [5–7,9,10]. The VKORC1 −1639 G > A genotype has the strongest association with low-dose warfarin requirement [5,7,9,10]. Our group has demonstrated that for the VKORC1 −1639 G > A genotype, patients with GG, GA, and AA genotypes had mean maintenance dose (SD) requirements of 6.7 (3.3), 4.2 (2.2), and 2.7 (1.2) mg/d, respectively [4]. As illustrated in Fig. 1, these dosage requirements corresponded with different therapeutic plasma S-warfarin concentrations. This was the first evidence of the mechanism-based effect of the VKORC1 −1639 G > A substitution leading to increased inhibition of this complex at lower S-warfarin concentrations when the −1639 A allele is present. These data reveal the target plasma S-warfarin concentration required to establish the target international normalized ratio (INR) response for each VKORC1 −1639 G > A genotype. This observation has been subsequently confirmed in an independent population of stabilized patients [11].

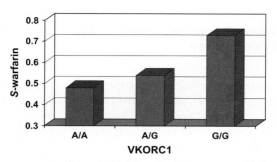

Fig. 1. Relationship between the VKORC1 −1639 G>A genotype, plasma *S*-warfarin concentration, and INR response. *S*-warfarin plasma concentrations at steady-state are graphed for each of the VKOR C1 −1639 G>A genotypes. All subjects were stabilized with an INR between 2.0 and 3.0. Mean dose (mg/d) and average plasma concentrations for each of the groups are as follows: VKORC1 −1639 AA (n = 8) 2.7 mg/d, 0.48 mg/L; VKOR C1 −1639 GA (n = 23) 4.3 mg/day, 0.54 mg/L; and VKOR C1 −1639 GG (n = 29) 6.7 mg/d, 0.73 mg/L. (*Data originally published in* Zhu Y, Shennan M, Reynolds KK, et al. Estimation of warfarin maintenance dose based on VKORC1 (−1639 G>A) and CYP2C9 genotypes. Clin Chem 2007;53(7):1199–205.)

CYP2C9 genotype and *S*-warfarin clearance

Cytochrome P450 2C9 (CYP2C9) metabolizes 80% to 85% of the more potent *S*-warfarin enantiomer to the inactive metabolites, 6- and 7-hydroxywarfarin. The CYP2C9 genotype accounts for 7.9% to 20.0% of the variance in maintenance dose requirement [4,7,8]. The primary pharmacokinetic consequence of CYP2C9 metabolic deficiency is a decreased *S*-warfarin clearance rate. CYP2C9*2 has anywhere from 12% to 70% and CYP2C9*3 has about 5% of the metabolic capacity of CYP2C9*1 [12,13]. Other variant alleles of CYP2C9 (*4, *5, *6, *8, *11) have been described but either occur in relatively lower frequencies (0.1% to 6%) or their frequencies have not been determined.

The *S*-warfarin clearance rate of an individual with the CYP2C9*1/*1 genotype is 39.6 L/h [14]. For the *2 allele, *S*-warfarin clearance decreases by 43% for individuals with a CYP2C9*1/*2 genotype and by 68% for individuals with a CYP2C9*2/*2 genotype [14]. For the *3 allele, *S*-warfarin clearance decreases by 48% for the CYP2C9*1/*3, and 91% for CYP2C9*3/*3 [14] genotypes. For the heterozygous CYP2C9*2/*3 genotype, *S*-warfarin clearances decrease by 77% [14].

VKORC1 and CYP2C9 genotype and ethnic prevalence

It has been demonstrated that 25% of dose variability could be explained by the patient's VKORC1 SNP haplotype, which shows a strong correlation with their warfarin dosage requirement (low-, intermediate-, and high-dose)

Table 1
VKORC1 genotype and ethnic prevalence [9,15,16]

VKORC1 −1639			VKORC1 1173		
Genotype	Caucasian	Asian	Genotype	Caucasian	African American
GG	39	3	CC	40.8	84.8
GA	47	18	CT	50.3	14.3
AA	14	78	TT	8.9	0.9

[6]. There is a strong correlation between ethnicity and VKORC1 SNP haplotype (Table 1). In general, African American populations have a higher proportion of individuals who require higher warfarin doses [6] than Caucasians. However, Asian populations have a higher proportion of individuals who require lower doses than Caucasians [6,15,16]. The CYP2C9 gene contains over 30 alleles, the most common of which is CYP2C9*1. The frequency of variant alleles differs depending on the ethnic diversity of the population. In general, African American and Asian populations have a larger percentage of CYP2C9*1 alleles than Caucasian populations (Table 2). Individuals with CYP2C9*1 alleles have the higher metabolic capacity when compared with patients with other CYP2C9 variant alleles.

Induction phase of treatment

Patients are at greatest risk for warfarin-induced adverse events during the induction phase [17,18]. Depending on patient cofactors, a typical induction strategy consists of a loading dose of 10 mg [19] or 5 mg [20,21], followed by dose adjustments based on INR values [2,5–7,9,11]. The higher loading dose will rapidly decrease anticoagulant protein C inducing a procoagulant effect [21,22]. To avoid this complication, heparin is often administered concurrently, during induction, until a therapeutic INR is reached. While the resemblance of the 5-mg induction dose to the maintenance dose may give the impression of being safer, it is not without its issues [23]. Just as with the 10-mg dose, a 5-mg induction dose can over anticoagulate some elderly patients [24–30], patients immediately following heart valve replacement [31–33], and those with inherited polymorphisms of CYP2C9 and VKORC1. A further drawback of the 5-mg loading

Table 2
CYP2C9 allelic frequency and ethnic prevalence

CYP2C9 Alleles	Caucasian, %	African American, %	Asian, %
*1	82.0	98.0	98.0
*2	12.0	3.0	0.0
*3	7.4	1.5	1.8

dose is that it may take longer to achieve a stable therapeutic INR [23] and patients remain on low molecular weight heparin longer than necessary. The protracted onset of anticoagulation increases the patient's risk of a thrombotic event.

International normalized ratio monitoring and interpretation

The INR measurement does not correlate with the antithrombotic activity of warfarin during the induction phase. The prolongation of the prothrombin time during the first 48 hours of therapy is largely achieved by the reduction of factor VII, which has the shortest elimination half-life (6 hours) of all vitamin K–dependent proteins. Further confounding the interpretation of INR during the induction phase, anticoagulant protein C also exhibits a similar half-life (9 hours) and reduction of this pool may induce a procoagulant effect in some warfarin-sensitive patients. The transient initial rise in INR attributable to the decrease in factor VII should not be interpreted as a stable measurement. The antithrombotic effects of warfarin do not become evident until pools of factors II and X are depleted. Depletion of factors II and X usually takes about 2 to 4 days.

After day 4, the INR measurement is less dependent on depletion of coagulation factors and is more dependent on inhibition of coagulation factor synthesis. Based on traditional pharmacologic principles, a dose response relationship must be evaluated in the context of steady state where medication concentration, over a dosing interval, is consistent for each subsequent dosage. The INR measurements reflect the true dose-response relationship once steady state is reached. At constant dosage, the forces that dictate the magnitude of S-warfarin plasma concentration and the rate of change of S-warfarin plasma concentration between doses, or steady state, are the pharmacokinetic parameters associated with CYP2C9 genotype. On average it will take individuals with the CYP2C9*1/*3 genotype 12 to 15 days after initiation of therapy or flowing dose adjustments for their INR to reflect steady state compared with individuals with the CYP2C9*1/*1 genotype who require 3 to 5 days (Fig. 2). Individuals with the CYP2C9*1/*2 genotype require an intermediate range of 6 to 9 days to reach steady state. Interpretation of the INR, during initiation or following dosage adjustments, without knowledge of time to reach steady state may lead to a possible overshoot of the target INR and place the patient at risk of hemorrhage or stroke.

Multivariate dose estimation equations

To shorten the time to reach therapeutic INR and to reduce the risk of over anticoagulation, dosing algorithms for the induction phase of therapy

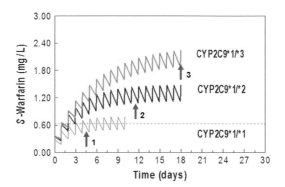

Fig. 2. Relationship between the rate of S-warfarin accumulation and approach to steady-state conditions and CYP2C9 genotype. This model represents the accumulation of plasma S-warfarin concentrations to steady state assuming repeated 5 mg/d dosing of average subjects keeping all other factors constant. Arrow # 1shows that patients with the CYP2C9 *1/*1 genotype reach steady state 3 to 5 days after initiation of therapy compared with arrow # 3, which shows that patients with the *1/*3 genotype reach steady state at about 12 to 15 days. Arrow # 2 shows that patients with the *1/*2 genotype require an intermediate time to reach steady state of 6 to 9 days. (*Adapted from* Linder MW, Looney S, Adams JE III, et al. Warfarin dose adjustments based on CYP2C9 genetic polymorphisms. J Thromb Thrombolysis 2002;14(3):227–32; with permission.)

were developed. The first of these was developed by Fennerty and colleagues [19], which has since been modified for patients immediately following heart-valve replacement [32], outpatient situations [34], and the elderly [27]. These algorithms were developed based on INR-response on day 4 following the initiation of warfarin therapy. These algorithms were further refined using patient cofactors (environmental, physical, and clinical) and made accessible through the development of computer-generated dosing regimens [35,36]. While these tools achieve better outcomes than trial-and-error dosing based on INR evaluation [35], they do not completely resolve issues of time to reach therapeutic INR or over anticoagulation [37].

Since the development of these tools, it has become widely accepted that genetic deficiencies of the CYP2C9 and VKORC1 genes are responsible for about 35% to 40% of dosing variability [5–7,38]. Using multiple regression analysis, the next generation of warfarin dosing models combined genetic factors with patient cofactors to predict maintenance dosing. Although not widely used in the clinical environment, several investigators have developed mathematical equations based on these genetic variants and other physical characteristics of the patient. These equations are typically capable of estimating the maintenance dose for a given patient to within 1 mg/day for approximately 50% of patients. Overall, the combination of both genetic and nongenetic factors, account for 50% to 60% of dosing variability [7,8,38–43].

To date, most attempts to prospectively apply CYP2C9 and VKORC1 genotyping to better manage warfarin therapy have limited the application of these test results in the context of associative multivariate equations. These equations take genetic and clinical factors into account to calculate an estimate of the eventual maintenance dose for a given patient [4,7,39,41,43–52]. Although the application of such equations has yielded some improvement in patient outcomes in a limited number of studies [44], they fail to provide clear and ongoing guidance for use of the information during the various stages of warfarin therapy.

Dynamic decision support tools

To present a dynamic approach to guiding warfarin therapy, based on S-warfarin clearance and plasma S-warfarin concentration at steady state (CaveSS) determined through CYP2C9 and VKORC1 genotyping and to take advantage of the progress made in genetics-based maintenance dose estimations, our group has developed a computational decision support tool (patent pending 60/859,803). Our tool combines genetic and clinical data to estimate warfarin dose and graphically displays progression of plasma S-warfarin concentrations approaching steady state with reference to the VKORC1-appropriate target CaveSS, thereby providing a time-based estimate of INR response. This approach also allows for calculation and modeling of loading strategies and is therefore able to provide guidance during the induction and transition dosing periods (time between induction and maintenance). Such modeling reduces the potential for INR misinterpretation and guides the appropriate timing of INR measurements based on time to reach steady state.

The accuracy of this tool for estimating maintenance dose requirement and in modeling the S-warfarin plasma concentrations has recently been reported [11]. Prospective trials of this novel technology are likely to demonstrate the advantage gained from ongoing application of the pharmacogenetic knowledge in terms of superior efficiency of the warfarin dose titration process.

Clinical scenarios

To illustrate how clinical decision support tools can be used to optimize patient care, a few clinical scenarios have been included. In current clinical practice, the results of pharmacogenetic testing are likely to be available at different times relative to the induction of warfarin therapy. For the hospitalized patient for whom warfarin therapy is anticipated, genotyping results can be made available before the patient receives the first dosage. In this clinical scenario, the pharmacogenetic test results can be useful in the design of the most appropriate induction dosing strategy. Based on the recent observation that the target therapeutic S-warfarin plasma concentration is governed by the VKORC1 genotype [4], a loading strategy to achieve this target plasma concentration can be determined by substituting the therapeutic plasma concentration for the patient's VKORC1 genotype into traditional loading dose calculations routinely used in clinical pharmacology (Fig. 3). Subsequently, the use of a multivariate equation incorporating both CYP2C9 and VKORC1 genotypes along with relevant clinical features of the patient allows for the maintenance dose to be estimated. By application of the appropriate S-warfarin clearance rate, determined by the CYP2C9 genotype, the time for repeated dosing to achieve steady-state plasma S-warfarin concentrations can be determined. This knowledge informs the practitioner of the time required for repeated dosing at the estimated maintenance dose to result in consistent S-warfarin concentrations to yield the most consistent and reliable INR response. INR measurements made under steady-state conditions most reliably reflect the

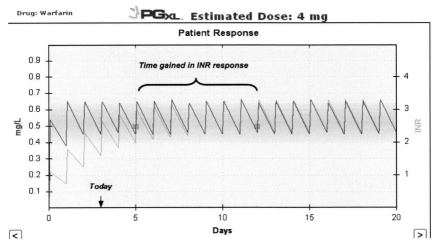

Fig. 3. Screen shot from a prototype clinical decision support tool. This figure illustrates the estimated dosage and S-warfarin plasma concentrations for a 58-year-old male of 175 lb having the CYP2C9 *1/*3 and VKOR C1 −1639 GA genotypes. Estimated maintenance dose was calculated based on the equation published by Zhu et al [4]. Plasma S-warfarin concentrations are shown for two dosing scenarios. The light blue line indicates repeated dosages of 4 mg/d. Note that this dosing strategy achieves steady state within the target therapeutic range of 0.4 to 0.63 mg/L as defined for the VKOR C1 GA genotype after approximately 8 to 9 days of therapy. The dark blue line illustrates the effects of inclusion of loading dose, calculated specifically for this patient's characteristics, which yields therapeutic concentrations within the first 2 days of therapy. The anticipated time to achieve a stable INR response for each dosing strategy is depicted by the gold boxes. Note that in the first scenario (light line), a therapeutic INR response is anticipated on day 12 of therapy, whereas in the loading scenario (dark line), the INR is anticipated to be reproducible and within the therapeutic range (2.0 to 3.0) by day 5 of therapy.

true dose-response relationship and provide the best guidance regarding the necessity for and magnitude of dosage adjustment.

A common scenario involves the urgent need for initiation of warfarin therapy before the availability of pharmacogenetic testing results. In this scenario, the practitioner must rely on traditional methods of warfarin initiation. However, upon the availability of CYP2C9 and VKORC1 genotyping results, the S-warfarin plasma concentration resulting from the past dosing history can be modeled. This model can then establish the current relationship between the target therapeutic concentration (determined by the patient's VKORC1 genotype) and the existing plasma concentration based on the past dosing history as well as the patient's CYP2C9 genotype-based S-warfarin clearance rate. At this point in time, the multivariate equation can be applied to estimating the maintenance dose for the patient, and a transition dosing strategy can be modeled to most quickly transition the current plasma S-warfarin concentration to the target therapeutic concentration. Further, the time to reach steady state under these revised dosing conditions can be determined from the CYP2C9 genotype and thereby guide the interpretation of subsequent INR measurements.

One further clinical scenario where a dynamic decision support tool may be of value is a scenario where maintenance warfarin therapy must be interrupted because of, for example, a pending surgical procedure (Fig. 4). In this scenario, modeling the change in plasma S-warfarin concentration reveals to the practitioner the period of time that warfarin therapy must be suspended to allow for restoration of baseline clotting potential of the patient. Further, upon re-initiation of therapy, a re-induction strategy can be developed by application of a similar strategy as that discussed for the loading dose scenario.

Future practice

These are but a few illustrations where the fundamental biochemical knowledge gained through CYP2C9 and VKORC1 genotyping can transcend the transient value gained through static, end point estimations of maintenance dose and yield a dynamic strategy for an efficient and reliable means of warfarin dosage titration. We anticipate that tools such as this will benefit a variety of professionals currently engaged in the support of patients prescribed warfarin. For example, a clinical laboratory, currently providing INR testing, could apply this technology to alert their clients when an INR measurement may not reflect a steady-state response thereby adding significant value to the INR testing service. Also, a clinical laboratory reporting CYP2C9 and VKORC1 test results could apply this technology to provide their clients with a means for sustained application of the pharmacogenetic test results throughout the patient's course of therapy. Coagulation clinic directors and PharmDs could dramatically improve the

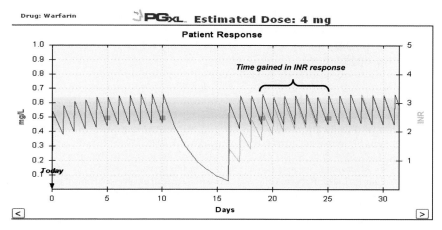

Fig. 4. Illustration of the application of PGx testing during long-term therapy. The scenario depicted is for the same patient characteristics as depicted in Fig. 3. In this situation, the patient has achieved a stable therapeutic response by day 10. However, this patient requires a surgical procedure and must not be anticoagulated at the time of the procedure. The clinical decision support tool can be used to model the number of days before the procedure that the warfarin dose should be withheld. In this case approximately 6 days is sufficient. Following the procedure, two re-initiation alternatives are demonstrated. The light line demonstrates the accumulation to steady state following an additional 9 days of dosing resulting in a therapeutic and reproducible INR response. In contrast, a re-loading strategy is depicted by the dark line, resulting in a therapeutic and reproducible restoration of the INR response within 3 days following the procedure.

efficiency of the clinic and improve the overall time in the therapeutic range by implementing this technology to guide dosing and monitoring decisions, and to educate patients of their individual characteristics which will influence their response to warfarin. We can envision researchers developing and testing novel hypotheses by applying this technology to gain deeper insight into the relationship between repeated warfarin dosing and INR response, identifying environmental factors that disrupt the concentration-response relationship, incorporating the quantitative and temporal effects of drug-drug interactions, and further defining the sources of inter- and intrapatient variability of warfarin response that contribute to the difficulty and risks associated with chronic warfarin therapy.

This approach may also have broader implications to the field of clinical pharmacogenetics and other disciplines where exposure-outcome relationships are dependent upon inherited factors and the cumulative effects of repeated exposures.

This tool illustrates an exciting evolution of the application of knowledge. The application of pharmacogenetic testing to warfarin therapy has proceeded through an evolution of application beginning with a categorical approach of dosage assignment based on CYP2C9 alone, followed by categorical assignment including VKORC1, proceeding to higher resolution assignment of dose based on multivariate equations, and ultimately to a dynamic and ongoing method to create a sustainable, highly individualized approach for application.

References

[1] Budnitz DS, Pollock DA, Weidenbach KN, et al. National surveillance of emergency department visits for outpatient adverse drug events. JAMA 2006;296(15):1858–66.

[2] Budnitz DS, Shehab N, Kegler SR, et al. Medication use leading to emergency department visits for adverse drug events in older adults. Ann Intern Med 2007;147(11):755–65.

[3] McWilliam A, Lutter R, Nardinelli C. Health care savings from personalizing medicine using genetic testing: the case of warfarin: AEI-Brookings Joint Center for Regulatory Studies; 2006.

[4] Zhu Y, Shennan M, Reynolds KK, et al. Estimation of warfarin maintenance dose based on VKORC1 (−1639 G>A) and CYP2C9 genotypes. Clin Chem 2007;53(7):1199–205.

[5] D'Andrea G, D'Ambrosio RL, Di Perna P, et al. A polymorphism in the VKORC1 gene is associated with an interindividual variability in the dose-anticoagulant effect of warfarin. Blood 2005;105(2):645–9.

[6] Rieder MJ, Reiner AP, Gage BF, et al. Effect of VKORC1 haplotypes on transcriptional regulation and warfarin dose. N Engl J Med 2005;352(22):2285–93.

[7] Sconce EA, Khan TI, Wynne HA, et al. The impact of CYP2C9 and VKORC1 genetic polymorphism and patient characteristics upon warfarin dose requirements: proposal for a new dosing regimen. Blood 2005;106(7):2329–33.

[8] Veenstra DL, You JH, Rieder MJ, et al. Association of vitamin K epoxide reductase complex 1 (VKORC1) variants with warfarin dose in a Hong Kong Chinese patient population. Pharmacogenet Genomics 2005;15(10):687–91.

[9] Yuan HY, Chen JJ, Lee MT, et al. A novel functional VKORC1 promoter polymorphism is associated with inter-individual and inter-ethnic differences in warfarin sensitivity. Hum Mol Genet 2005;14(13):1745–51.

[10] Bodin L, Verstuyft C, Tregouet DA, et al. Cytochrome P450 2C9 (CYP2C9) and vitamin K epoxide reductase (VKORC1) genotypes as determinants of acenocoumarol sensitivity. Blood 2005;106(1):135–40.

[11] Reynolds KK, Gage BF, Silvestrov NA, et al. Accuracy of genotype-based warfarin dose estimation and plasma S-warfarin pharmacokinetic modeling. Paper presented at the American Association of Clinical Chemistry Annual Meeting. Washington, DC; 2008.

[12] Takahashi H, Echizen H. Pharmacogenetics of warfarin elimination and its clinical implications. Clin Pharmacokinet 2001;40(8):587–603.

[13] Kirchheiner J, Brockmoller J. Clinical consequences of cytochrome P450 2C9 polymorphisms. Clin Pharmacol Ther 2005;77(1):1–16.

[14] Scordo MG, Pengo V, Spina E, et al. Influence of CYP2C9 and CYP2C19 genetic polymorphisms on warfarin maintenance dose and metabolic clearance. Clin Pharmacol Ther 2002; 72(6):702–10.

[15] Schelleman H, Chen Z, Kealey C, et al. Warfarin response and vitamin K epoxide reductase complex 1 in African Americans and Caucasians. Clin Pharmacol Ther 2007; 81(5):742–7.

[16] Schelleman H, Limdi NA, Kimmel SE. Ethnic differences in warfarin maintenance dose requirement and its relationship with genetics. Pharmacogenomics 2008;9(9):1331–46.

[17] Fihn SD, McDonell M, Martin D, et al. Risk factors for complications of chronic anticoagulation. A multicenter study. Warfarin Optimized Outpatient Follow-up Study Group. Ann Intern Med 1993;118(7):511–20.

[18] Landefeld CS, Beyth RJ. Anticoagulant-related bleeding: clinical epidemiology, prediction, and prevention. Am J Med 1993;95(3):315–28.

[19] Fennerty A, Dolben J, Thomas P, et al. Flexible induction dose regimen for warfarin and prediction of maintenance dose. Br Med J (Clin Res Ed) 1984;288(6426):1268–70.

[20] Tait RC, Sefcick A. A warfarin induction regimen for out-patient anticoagulation in patients with atrial fibrillation. Br J Haematol 1998;101(3):450–4.

[21] Harrison L, Johnston M, Massicotte MP, et al. Comparison of 5-mg and 10-mg loading doses in initiation of warfarin therapy. Ann Intern Med 1997;126(2):133–6.

[22] Vigano S, Mannucci PM, Solinas S, et al. Decrease in protein C antigen and formation of an abnormal protein soon after starting oral anticoagulant therapy. Br J Haematol 1984;57(2): 213–20.

[23] Harper P, Monahan K, Baker B. Warfarin induction at 5 mg daily is safe with a low risk of anticoagulant overdose: results of an audit of patients with deep vein thrombosis commencing warfarin. Intern Med J 2005;35(12):717–20.

[24] Ansell J, Hirsh J, Poller L, et al. The pharmacology and management of the vitamin K antagonists: the Seventh ACCP Conference on Antithrombotic and Thrombolytic Therapy. Chest 2004;126(3 Suppl):204S–33S.

[25] Cooper MW, Hendra TJ. Prospective evaluation of a modified Fennerty regimen for anticoagulating elderly people. Age Ageing 1998;27(5):655–6.

[26] Garcia D, Regan S, Crowther M, et al. Warfarin maintenance dosing patterns in clinical practice: implications for safer anticoagulation in the elderly population. Chest 2005; 127(6):2049–56.

[27] Gedge J, Orme S, Hampton KK, et al. A comparison of a low-dose warfarin induction regimen with the modified Fennerty regimen in elderly inpatients. Age Ageing 2000;29(1):31–4.

[28] O'Connell MB, Kowal PR, Allivato CJ, et al. Evaluation of warfarin initiation regimens in elderly inpatients. Pharmacotherapy 2000;20(8):923–30.

[29] Roberts GW, Druskeit T, Jorgensen LE, et al. Comparison of an age adjusted warfarin loading protocol with empirical dosing and Fennerty's protocol. Aust N Z J Med 1999;29(5): 731–6.

[30] Siguret V, Gouin I, Debray M, et al. Initiation of warfarin therapy in elderly medical inpatients: a safe and accurate regimen. Am J Med 2005;118(2):137–42.

[31] Lee SY, Nam MH, Kim JS, et al. A case report of a patient carrying CYP2C9*3/4 genotype with extremely low warfarin dose requirement. J Korean Med Sci 2007;22(3):557–9.

[32] Ageno W, Turpie AG, Steidl L, et al. Comparison of a daily fixed 2.5-mg warfarin dose with a 5-mg, international normalized ratio adjusted, warfarin dose initially following heart valve replacement. Am J Cardiol 2001;88(1):40–4.

[33] Rahman M, BinEsmael TM, Payne N, et al. Increased sensitivity to warfarin after heart valve replacement. Ann Pharmacother 2006;40(3):397–401.

[34] Oates A, Jackson PR, Austin CA, et al. A new regimen for starting warfarin therapy in out-patients. Br J Clin Pharmacol 1998;46(2):157–61.

[35] Poller L, Shiach CR, MacCallum PK, et al. Multicentre randomised study of computerised anticoagulant dosage. European Concerted Action on Anticoagulation. Lancet 1998; 352(9139):1505–9.

[36] Ageno W, Johnson J, Nowacki B, et al. A computer generated induction system for hospitalized patients starting on oral anticoagulant therapy. Thromb Haemost 2000;83(6): 849–52.

[37] Vadher BD, Patterson DL, Leaning MS. Validation of an algorithm for oral anticoagulant dosing and appointment scheduling. Clin Lab Haematol 1995;17(4):339–45.

[38] Wadelius M, Chen LY, Downes K, et al. Common VKORC1 and GGCX polymorphisms associated with warfarin dose. Pharmacogenomics J 2005;5(4):262–70.

[39] Kimura R, Miyashita K, Kokubo Y, et al. Genotypes of vitamin K epoxide reductase, gamma-glutamyl carboxylase, and cytochrome P450 2C9 as determinants of daily warfarin dose in Japanese patients. Thromb Res 2007;120(2):181–6.

[40] Shikata E, Ieiri I, Ishiguro S, et al. Multiple gene polymorphisms and warfarin sensitivity. Eur J Clin Pharmacol 2006;62(10):881–3.

[41] Tham LS, Goh BC, Nafziger A, et al. A warfarin-dosing model in Asians that uses single-nucleotide polymorphisms in vitamin K epoxide reductase complex and cytochrome P450 2C9. Clin Pharmacol Ther 2006;80(4):346–55.

[42] Vecsler M, Loebstein R, Almog S, et al. Combined genetic profiles of components and regulators of the vitamin K-dependent gamma-carboxylation system affect individual sensitivity to warfarin. Thromb Haemost 2006;95(2):205–11.

[43] Wadelius M, Chen LY, Eriksson N, et al. Association of warfarin dose with genes involved in its action and metabolism. Hum Genet 2007;121(1):23–34.

[44] Anderson JL, Horne BD, Stevens SM, et al. Randomized trial of genotype-guided versus standard warfarin dosing in patients initiating oral anticoagulation. Circulation 2007; 116(22):2563–70.

[45] Caldwell MD, Berg RL, Zhang KQ, et al. Evaluation of genetic factors for warfarin dose prediction. Clin Med Res 2007;5(1):8–16.

[46] Carlquist JF, Horne BD, Muhlestein JB, et al. Genotypes of the cytochrome p450 isoform, CYP2C9, and the vitamin K epoxide reductase complex subunit 1 conjointly determine stable warfarin dose: a prospective study. J Thromb Thrombolysis 2006;22(3):191–7.

[47] Gage B, Eby C, Johnson J, et al. Use of pharmacogenetic and clinical factors to predict the therapeutic dose of warfarin. Clin Pharmacol Ther 2008;84:326–31.

[48] Gage BF, Eby C, Milligan PE, et al. Use of pharmacogenetics and clinical factors to predict the maintenance dose of warfarin. Thromb Haemost 2004;91(1):87–94.

[49] Herman D, Locatelli I, Grabnar I, et al. Influence of CYP2C9 polymorphisms, demographic factors and concomitant drug therapy on warfarin metabolism and maintenance dose. Pharmacogenomics J 2005;5(3):193–202.

[50] Miao L, Yang J, Huang C, et al. Contribution of age, body weight, and CYP2C9 and VKORC1 genotype to the anticoagulant response to warfarin: proposal for a new dosing regimen in Chinese patients. Eur J Clin Pharmacol 2007;63(12):1135–41.

[51] Voora D, Eby C, Linder MW, et al. Prospective dosing of warfarin based on cytochrome P-450 2C9 genotype. Thromb Haemost 2005;93(4):700–5.

[52] Wen MS, Lee M, Chen JJ, et al. Prospective study of warfarin dosage requirements based on CYP2C9 and VKORC1 genotypes. Clin Pharmacol Ther 2008;84:83–9.

ELSEVIER
SAUNDERS

CLINICS IN
LABORATORY
MEDICINE

Clin Lab Med 28 (2008) 553–567

Pharmacogenomics of Tamoxifen and Irinotecan Therapies

Alicia Algeciras-Schimnich, PhD[a],
Dennis J. O'Kane, PhD[b],
Christine L.H. Snozek, PhD[a],*

[a]*Division of Clinical Biochemistry and Immunology, Department of Laboratory Medicine and Pathology, College of Medicine, Hilton 730, Mayo Clinic, 200 1st Street Southwest, Rochester, MN 55905, USA*
[b]*Division of Clinical Biochemistry and Immunology, Department of Laboratory Medicine and Pathology, College of Medicine, Hilton 410, Mayo Clinic, 200 1st Street Southwest, Rochester, MN 55905, USA*

Optimizing treatment of malignancies requires determining not only which therapeutic agents are preferable for a given tumor type but also defining which patients will benefit from administration of a given therapy. Recently, notable improvements in the targeted therapy of cancer have come about as a result of the growing recognition of the role that inherited variability in enzymatic activity plays in drug metabolism and efficacy. Genotypic information can be used to enhance several aspects of therapeutic optimization, from selecting the patient population most likely to benefit from a particular agent to predicting which patients are predisposed to adverse drug responses. This article discusses the application of pharmacogenetics to oncology in the context of the chemotherapeutics irinotecan and tamoxifen.

Irinotecan therapy in colorectal cancer

Irinotecan (Camptosar, CPT-11) is a camptothecin-derived topoisomerase I inhibitor approved by the Food and Drug Administration (FDA) for use in metastatic colorectal cancer, either as a first-line component of combined therapy, or as a second-line single-agent treatment [1]. It is also currently in clinical trials for use in various other solid tumors [2]. When

---

* Corresponding author.
E-mail address: hattrup.christine@mayo.edu (C.L.H. Snozek).

used in first-line combination therapy (eg, with 5′-fluorouracil [5′-FU] and leucovorin in the FOLFIRI regimen), irinotecan is infused either at a high dose every 3 weeks, or fractionated into lower doses for weekly treatments. As a single agent for treatment of 5′-FU–refractory colorectal cancer, irinotecan is given either weekly or biweekly. Recommended doses range from 50 to 350 mg/m^2 body surface area, depending on the specific regimen and dosing schedule [1].

Although irinotecan is an active cytotoxic agent, most of the administered dose is converted by carboxylesterase enzymes to its more potent metabolite, SN-38. This conversion is inefficient in vivo, and is a potential target area for improvements in irinotecan delivery [3]. Irinotecan and SN-38 can be metabolized by several cytochrome P450 (CYP) enzymes to inactive compounds, although these represent minor pathways of biotransformation [4]. However, inhibition of CYP3A4 by irinotecan and SN-38 may be a concern for patients treated concurrently with other drugs that are CYP3A4 substrates.

Adverse responses to irinotecan can occur immediately after administration or after a delay [1]. Early toxicity manifests as diarrhea that can be accompanied by other cholinergic symptoms (eg, rhinitis, lacrimation, diaphoresis); this response generally occurs after administration of an anticholinergic agent such as atropine. Late-onset toxicity occurs more than 24 hours after administration and most commonly consists of prolonged diarrhea or marked neutropenia (grade 3/4), either of which can be life threatening [5]. Severe toxicity correlates, in general, to SN-38 exposure, as determined by the area under the time-concentration curve (AUC) [6].

Uridine diphosphate-glucuronyltransferase 1A1 polymorphisms and irinotecan toxicity

The major route of irinotecan excretion is facilitated by conversion to SN-38 followed by glucuronidation of the metabolite (SN-38-G) [7]. The enzyme primarily responsible for this latter step is uridine diphosphate-glucuronyltransferase (UGT) 1A1 (UGT1A1). The UGT1A gene locus actually encodes for at least nine related proteins; each family member has a unique exon 1 and all share the common exons 2 to 5 [8]. UGT1A1 is the best characterized of these enzymes, largely because of the mild (Gilbert) and severe (Crigler-Najjar) syndromes of unconjugated hyperbilirubinemia associated with reduced UGT1A1 activity.

Lower expression of UGT1A1 results in prolonged exposure of patients to the active compound SN-38, increasing the risk for toxicity [9]. The most common genetic cause of reduced UGT1A1 activity is a polymorphism in the promoter TATA box, resulting in seven thymine-adenine repeats in contrast to the six repeats present in the wild-type allele [8]. This seven-repeat allele, named UGT1A1*28, is associated with lower transcription of UGT1A1 and has a homozygous frequency of approximately 10% in

Caucasians and 20% in African Americans. Two other, less-prevalent TATA box variants, termed UGT1A1*36 and *37, have been described, with five and eight TA repeats, respectively [10]. Transcription appears to vary inversely with the number of TA repeats; thus, UGT1A1*36 shows equivalent or enhanced expression compared with wild type, whereas UGT1A1*37 produces lower enzyme levels than even the UGT1A1*28 variant [11]. Although studies to date are limited, the eight-repeat allele (found primarily in African Americans) would be expected to show comparable or higher risk for irinotecan toxicity than that seen for UGT1A1*28 patients.

In 2004, recognition of studies linking the homozygous UGT1A1*28 genotype to increased risk for severe toxicity led the FDA to recommend modifying the irinotecan package insert to suggest reduced dosage for patients who have the variant genotype [5,12]. Shortly thereafter, a rapid testing kit was approved for identification of *28/*28 patients (Invader UGT1A1, Third Wave Technologies, Madison, Wisconsin). The *28/*28 genotype is a significant predictor of toxicity, although less reliable than direct measurement of the SN-38 AUC [6]. However, it is clear that UGT1A1*28 is not the only allele capable of reducing the clearance of SN-38; in addition to TATA box variants, several missense polymorphisms are common, notably in Asian populations [13]. Neither the irinotecan package insert nor the FDA-approved assay addresses these variants, despite in vitro and in vivo evidence that SN-38 glucuronidation is impaired.

UGT1A1*6, encoding a glutamine to arginine mutation at residue 71 (G71R), is found in roughly 20% of Asians and is likely a major source of irinotecan toxicity in this group [14]. The ability of this variant to form SN-38-G in vitro is approximately half that of the wild-type protein, providing a mechanism for the increased exposure to SN-38 reported in patients who have the UGT1A1*6 genotype [15,16]. The UGT1A1*27 (P229Q) allele is a less common variant found in 3% of Asians; it has comparable glucuronidating activity to UGT1A1*6. A third missense mutation in Asians is UGT1A1*7 (Y486D), which produces a severe decrease in function, resulting in a Crigler-Najjar type II syndrome in the homozygous state [15]. The UGT1A1*7 allele is rare but, in the heterozygous state, would be predicted to result in a risk for irinotecan toxicity comparable to homozygosity for the more prevalent UGT1A1 variant alleles.

One key issue that is as yet unresolved is whether a genetic predisposition to impaired SN-38 glucuronidation necessarily enhances the risk for toxicity. Although it is recognized that homozygous UGT1A1*28 patients are more likely, but not guaranteed, to be intolerant of irinotecan, a recent metareview by Hoskins and colleagues [17] has suggested that the risk for severe neutropenia associated with the *28/*28 genotype depends on the specific drug regimen studied. High-dose irinotecan (>250 mg/m^2, given every 3 weeks) was indeed associated with a much higher odds ratios for developing neutropenia in homozygous *28/*28 patients. In contrast, low-dose regimens (<150 mg/m^2, given weekly) were not associated with significantly increased toxicity in patients who had the variant genotype, suggesting that the effect of UGT1A1 genetics might depend on the amount of irinotecan given. Severe diarrhea did not show an association with irinotecan dose. These findings are in agreement with pediatric studies in which irinotecan was given in low doses over multiple days within a 7- to 14-day window, and which showed minimal association of the *28/*28 genotype with hematologic toxicity [18,19].

The influence of dose and dosing schedule on toxicity suggests that recommended irinotecan dose modifications might need to be tailored to each particular regimen, especially with respect to combination therapies. However, prospective studies addressing the question of optimal irinotecan dosing for UGT1A1-deficient patients are lacking. Hoskins and colleagues [17] found that biweekly, moderate-dose regimens showed an intermediate elevation in risk for neutropenia in *28/*28 patients, suggesting that, although dose reduction is an appropriate option in such regimens, the degree to which risk for toxicity is enhanced might be acceptable to some patients and clinicians. Given the success of moderate levels of irinotecan in combination with various other therapeutic agents [20], it is possible that patients who have impaired UGT1A1 function may still benefit from the full dose of irinotecan in biweekly regimens, if careful selection of therapeutic options is made according to individual tolerance for risk.

The association of toxicity with reduced SN-38 glucuronidation suggests that those patients who have wild-type or enhanced UGT1A1 activity may well tolerate higher doses of irinotecan. Enhanced excretion after glucuronidation has been linked to the resistance of colorectal cancer cells to cytotoxic agents [21], suggesting that insufficient exposure to SN-38 is a possible mechanism for irinotecan therapeutic failure in patients who have adequate UGT activity. Because initial dose recommendations were established using patient populations who had mixed UGT1A1 genotypes, it is to be hoped that dose-escalation trials will determine whether patients who have wild-type UGT1A1 activity (ie, *1/*1 genotype) are benefited by, and are able to tolerate, higher levels of irinotecan than those currently recommended [22].

Other uridine diphosphate-glucuronyltransferase 1A enzymes

In addition to UGT1A1, UGT family members 1A7, 1A9, and 1A10 have all been shown to glucuronidate SN-38 in vitro, indicating that alterations in the activity of any of these enzymes could potentially affect irinotecan efficacy and toxicity [8]. UGT1A7 is largely expressed in the esophagus and stomach, whereas UGT1A9, like UGT1A1, is found predominantly in the liver and lower gastrointestinal tract. In vitro, UGT1A9 variants display considerably reduced glucuronidation of SN-38 [23]. However, the few in vivo studies of the influence of UGT1A9 on SN-38 metabolism suggest that these variants are rare in European populations and have a limited effect on irinotecan pharmacokinetics [24].

In contrast, UGT1A7 variant alleles are common; in vitro, several result in decreased SN-38 glucuronidation [8]. The limited clinical studies of this gene have shown either negligible influence on response to irinotecan [25], or a surprising reduction in diarrhea combined with enhanced antitumor response for those UGT1A7 variants with reduced in vitro activity [26]. If these results are repeated by other groups, additional work will be required to clarify how a protein not normally expressed in colonic tissue affects the response of colorectal tumors to chemotherapy. A small Japanese study found that low-activity polymorphisms in UGT1A7 and UGT1A9 were linked to the common UGT1A1*6 variant, suggesting that haplotype analysis may provide information regarding clinically significant alterations in several UGT genes [27]. Unique variants and different allele frequencies have been described for UGT1A7 in African Americans [23], indicating that this population specifically should be included in further studies of the role of UGT1A7 in irinotecan pharmacokinetics.

Future directions

Given the existence of multiple enzymes potentially involved in SN-38 glucuronidation, each with several variant alleles, prospective clinical trials involving comprehensive UGT genotyping and careful attention to dose and dosing schedule are advisable. Development of various rapid assays [28] for the UGT1A1*28/*28 genotype have facilitated study of this allele; these methods are being extended to include further characterization of the TATA box [29] and UGT1A1 coding sequence [30] to better span the range of clinically relevant polymorphisms. At the same time, improvements in delivery [31] and activation [3] of irinotecan are being introduced, and use of this drug is expanding well beyond the realm of colorectal cancer. Advancements in these areas are to be welcomed but highlight the need to clarify issues regarding genetic influences on metabolism and elimination. Ready access to genotypic information will undoubtedly further understanding of the effects of UGT family members on irinotecan disposition in vivo, allowing better individualized tailoring of this therapeutic agent to its recipients.

In contrast to UGT1A-related irinotecan toxicity, where low enzyme activity results in prolonged exposure to a toxic metabolite, another common chemotherapeutic agent, tamoxifen, has received recent attention for the role of specific enzymes in conversion of this prodrug to its active metabolites. The second part of this article discusses the effects of CYP variants on tamoxifen therapy.

Tamoxifen therapy in breast cancer

Tamoxifen, a selective estrogen receptor (ER) modulator, is approved by the FDA for the treatment and prevention of breast cancer [32,33]. A meta-analysis of tamoxifen therapy trials showed that, in patients who had ER-positive breast cancer, administration of tamoxifen as adjuvant therapy for 5 years following anthracycline-based chemotherapy reduced the recurrence rate by nearly 50% and the mortality rate by a third after 15 years of follow-up [34]. However, treatment with tamoxifen is not without challenges. The most common side effect of tamoxifen therapy is hot flashes; the most severe adverse effects are the reported incidence of endometrial cancer and thromboembolic events [32]. Despite the life-threatening nature of these events, the overall therapeutic benefit of tamoxifen in certain populations outweighs the potential risks associated with long-term therapy.

Tamoxifen metabolism

The antitumor effects of tamoxifen are mediated by its antiestrogen activity. Tamoxifen binds the ER and blocks the action of estrogen, a hormone that stimulates the growth of some cells types, including malignant cells [35]. Tamoxifen is considered a prodrug and requires extensive metabolism to elicit its antitumor effects. Tamoxifen is metabolized in the liver primarily by the enzymes CYP2D6, CYP3A4, and CYP3A5. The major metabolites of tamoxifen include N-desmethyl-tamoxifen (NDT), 4-hydroxy-tamoxifen (4-OH-TAM), and 4-hydroxy-N-desmethyltamoxifen (endoxifen) (Fig. 1) [36–40]. NDT is produced by CYP3A4/5-mediated demethylation of tamoxifen and accounts for approximately 90% of the parent drug [40]. In contrast, 4-OH-TAM, generated by various CYP enzymes, including CYP2D6 [41], constitutes less than 10% of total tamoxifen metabolites but has a 100-fold greater affinity for the ER and is 30 to 100 fold more potent than tamoxifen in suppressing estrogen-dependent cell proliferation [42–44].

For many years, 4-OH-TAM was considered the main active metabolite of tamoxifen. Currently, however, endoxifen is believed to be the tamoxifen metabolite responsible for the antitumor effects. Endoxifen is metabolized from NDT by CYP2D6 [40]. It was originally identified in 1989 [37] but only recently shown to be as potent as 4-OH-TAM in inhibiting estrogen-mediated cell proliferation in vitro and to be present in concentrations 6 to 10 fold higher than 4-OH-TAM [39,45,46]. Because endoxifen generation primarily depends on CYP2D6 activity, genetic variants of CYP2D6 and drugs that modulate the activity of CYP2D6 could have a significant impact on the therapeutic outcome of tamoxifen-treated patients. In addition, the altered enzyme activity of CYP2D6 conferred by gene polymorphisms likely explains a portion of the large interindividual variation observed in response to tamoxifen treatment.

Cytochrome P450 2D6 polymorphisms and tamoxifen treatment

CYP2D6 plays an important role in the phase I metabolism of 25% of drugs on the market, including beta-blockers, antidepressants, antiarrythmics,

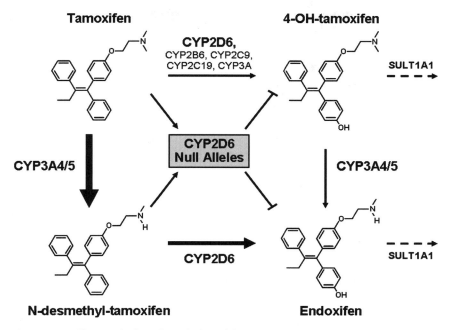

Fig. 1. Tamoxifen metabolism. CYP3A4/5 and CYP2D6 are the main CYP enzymes involved in the metabolism of tamoxifen. CYP3A4/5 mediates the generation of NDT, the major metabolite, whereas CYP2D6 is involved in the generation of 4-OH-TAM, a minor metabolite. NDT and 4-OH-TAM are further metabolized to the active metabolite endoxifen by CYP2D6 and CYP3A4/5, respectively. In patients who have CYP2D6 null alleles, the metabolism of tamoxifen is blocked, preventing generation of 4-OH-TAM and endoxifen. Other CYP enzymes, including CYP2B6, CYP2C9, and CYP2C19, appear to play a small role in the metabolism of tamoxifen. Sulfation mediated by sulfotransferase 1A1 (SULT1A1) plays a role in tamoxifen metabolite clearance.

antipsychotics, and anticancer drugs [47,48]. CYP2D6 activity is highly variable in the population as a result of polymorphisms in the CYP2D6 gene. Currently, at least 68 CYP2D6 gene variants have been described (www.cypalleles.ki.se) that can be grouped phenotypically into poor (PM), intermediate (IM), extensive (EM), and ultrarapid (UM) metabolizers. The frequency of these phenotypes varies widely among ethnic groups. For example, CYP2D6*4, one of the most important alleles in conferring a PM phenotype, accounts for 12% to 21% of northern European populations but only 1% to 2% of Asians and Black Africans [48]. Some of the most important allelic variants of 2D6 include the wild-type allele CYP2D6*1, which encodes for a fully functional enzyme; alleles associated with no enzymatic activity (CYP2D6*3–*8, *11–*16, *18–*20, *38, *40, *42, *44) or reduced activity (CYP2D6*9, *10, *17, *29, *36, *37, *41); and the alleles in which multiple copies of the CYP2D6 gene (*2, *4, *10, *17, *35, *41) have been reported.

Analysis of tamoxifen metabolism and CYP2D6 genotype in women undergoing tamoxifen treatment demonstrated that patients who have two or more functional alleles of CYP2D6*1 have a higher concentration of endoxifen in plasma compared with patients who have one or more non-functional alleles, including CYP2D6*3 to *6 [49]. The endoxifen levels were also lower in patients who had two functional alleles, who were taking known CYP2D6 inhibitors, indicating that reduced CYP2D6 activity results in impaired metabolism of tamoxifen. A more comprehensive analysis of genotype in relation to endoxifen levels was conducted by Borges and colleagues [50], wherein 158 patients across multiple ethnic populations had CYP2D6 genotype and endoxifen plasma concentrations analyzed. Null alleles (CYP2D6*3, *4, *5, *6), dysfunctional alleles (CYP2D6*9, *10, *17, *29, *41), and functional alleles (CYP2D6*1, *2, *35) were identified in these patients. The study demonstrated that individuals considered to have IM, based on genotype (eg, heterozygotes for the *10 [reduced activity] or *4 [no activity] alleles), had similar concentrations of endoxifen to those considered to have PM. In addition, patients who had a UM phenotype had a higher concentration of endoxifen compared with those who had EM. This study further strengthens the hypothesis that CYP2D6 genotyping provides a good prediction of endoxifen concentration in the plasma of patients who have breast cancer and are treated with tamoxifen.

The role of CYP2D6 genetic variants in the treatment outcome of patients taking tamoxifen was analyzed retrospectively in 223 postmenopausal women enrolled in the North Central Cancer Treatment Group trial [51]. In this study, two variants of CYP2D6 were examined, *4 (the most common null allele contributing to the PM state) and *6 (an infrequent PM allele). Women who had the CYP2D6*4/*4 genotype had shorter relapse-free time and worse disease-free survival compared with women who had either one or no *4 alleles. In addition, none of the women who had the CYP2D6*4/*4 genotype experienced moderate or severe hot flashes, compared with 20% of the women who had a CYP2D6*4/*1 or CYP2D6*1/*1 genotype. An Italian tamoxifen chemoprevention trial also reported that patients who developed breast cancer (ie, failed chemopreventive therapy) were significantly more likely to have the CYP2D6*4/*4 genotype [52]. Borges and colleagues [50] expanded these findings by analyzing the effect of 33 different CYP2D6 variants: tamoxifen-treated patients carrying the CYP2D6 alleles *4, *5, *10, *41, all associated with impaired formation of the active tamoxifen metabolites, had significantly higher recurrence rates, shorter relapse-free periods, and worse event-free survival rates when compared with carriers of functional alleles. All together, these studies suggest that women carrying CYP2D6 alleles with null or decreased activity are less likely to benefit from tamoxifen treatment.

However, two other groups have reported different outcomes between CYP2D6 genotype and tamoxifen treatment [53–55]. Nowell and colleagues [53] found no association between CYP2D6*4 genotype and overall survival in a retrospective cohort of 162 patients treated with tamoxifen. Additionally, Wegman and colleagues [54,55] demonstrated that patients homozygous or heterozygous for the CYP2D6*4 allele (n = 32) had better disease-free survival than patients who did not have the *4 allele (n = 79), although the differences were not statistically significant. The reasons for these discrepancies are not clear at this time, although several factors have been suggested [56].

Cytochrome P450 2D6 inhibitors during tamoxifen treatment

Hot flashes are one of the most common side effects of tamoxifen treatment [32]. Antidepressants, such as the selective serotonin reuptake inhibitors (SSRI), are commonly coadministered with tamoxifen to alleviate this side effect. However, it has been demonstrated that coadministration of paroxetine or fluoxetine (two SSRI and potent inhibitors of CYP2D6) in patients carrying an EM phenotype results in a significant reduction of endoxifen levels when compared with EM patients not using CYP2D6 inhibitors [49,50]. In contrast, weak inhibitors of CYP2D6, such as venlafaxine, did not show a statistically significant reduction of endoxifen levels when compared with patients not taking inhibitors [49]. A recent study by Goetz and colleagues [57] assessed the combined effect of genetic variation and drug-induced inhibition of CYP2D6 on breast cancer outcomes. In this analysis, 226 patients were segregated according to whether potent or weak/moderate CYP2D6 inhibitors were coprescribed with tamoxifen. Based on the genotype and medication history, patients were classified as having an extensive (normal) or decreased CYP2D6 metabolism. Patients who had decreased metabolism had significantly shorter time to recurrence and worse relapse-free survival than patients who had extensive metabolism. All together, these studies indicate that coadministration of potent CYP2D6 inhibitors should be avoided in patients taking tamoxifen because they might jeopardize the success of the treatment. In patients who have hot flashes, venlafaxine is a potential therapy because it does not significantly affect the levels of endoxifen and has been shown to be effective in the treatment of hot flashes in breast cancer patients [49,58].

Food and drug administration recommendations on tamoxifen

In October 2006, an FDA advisory panel met to discuss the current evidence regarding CYP2D6 genotyping and tamoxifen treatment outcomes [59]. The panel agreed that the labeling for tamoxifen should be revised to alert physicians that patients who have breast cancer and are CYP2D6 PM have an increased risk for cancer recurrence. In addition, the panel agreed that the package insert should warn that SSRI can inhibit the ability of CYP2D6 to metabolize tamoxifen. Although the panel agreed that information about the availability of genotyping should be included on the revised labeling, a consensus was not reached as to whether testing should be an option or a requirement.

Cytochrome P450 2D6 genotyping and tamoxifen treatment: clinical practice

The limited information available on current practice indicates that physicians are informing patients of the importance of CYP2D6 genotyping in tamoxifen treatment outcomes, and are also discouraging the coadministration of tamoxifen and potent inhibitors of CYP2D6 [56]. Knowledge of patient genotype is useful in situations where an alternative therapy is available. Review of a limited number of patients in which CYP2D6 genotyping has been performed in the authors' institution showed that PMs are being prescribed aromatase inhibitors instead of tamoxifen.

Aromatase inhibitors block the enzyme aromatase, involved in the conversion of androgens to estrogen, thereby lowering the estrogen concentration in postmenopausal women. Aromatase inhibitors have become an accepted therapy for postmenopausal women who have breast cancer because the results of randomized clinical trials have demonstrated superior efficacy and better overall safety compared with tamoxifen [60]. With respect to breast cancer prevention, raloxifene might be an alternative therapy for CYP2D6 PM. Raloxifene, a selective ER modulator, has been approved by the FDA for reducing the risk for invasive breast cancer in postmenopausal women who have osteoporosis or are at high risk for developing breast cancer. Raloxifene has been shown to be as effective as tamoxifen in reducing the incidence of breast cancer in postmenopausal women at high risk for developing breast cancer [61,62].

Role of other polymorphisms in tamoxifen treatment outcome

The influence of allelic variants of CYP3A, CYP2C9, CYP2C19, and sulfotransferase 1A1 (SULT1A1) has also been studied. CYP3A4/5 is involved in the conversion of tamoxifen to NDT [40], but determining the role of CYP3A5 polymorphisms in tamoxifen treatment outcome is controversial. Patients who have breast cancer and the CYP3A5*3 polymorphism, which results in a truncated nonfunctional protein, showed no statistically significant difference in the plasma concentrations of tamoxifen or its metabolites [49,63]. With respect to patient outcomes, no differences in time to relapse, disease-free survival, or overall survival have been observed in the CYP3A5*3 genotype group [51]. Wegman and colleagues [54] recently reported that patients homozygous for CYP3A5*3 have an improved recurrence-free survival. These results are unexpected because this genotype represents an inactive form of the enzyme and should therefore not catalyze the formation of NDT, the precursor of endoxifen. However, it has been suggested that CYP3A5 is a minor contributor to the overall metabolism of

CYP3A, when compared with CYP3A4 [64,65]. Currently, no published studies have investigated the influence of CYP3A4 polymorphisms on tamoxifen treatment outcomes.

CYP2C9 and CYP2C19 are, to a lesser extent, involved in the formation of NDT [38,40,41]. Schroth and colleagues [66] investigated the influence of the CYP2C19 variants *2, *3, and *17 in tamoxifen treatment outcome. Patients who had the UM allele, CYP2C19*17, had a more favorable outcome with a lower risk for relapse and prolonged relapse-free time when compared with patients who had the wild-type *1 allele. The two null variants *2 and *3 showed no differences in treatment outcome compared with the *1 allele. In contrast, variants of CYP2C9 with decreased enzyme activity (*2 and *3) did not affect the levels of tamoxifen metabolites or treatment outcomes, when compared with patients carrying the wild-type allele [49,66].

SULT1A1 is involved in the sulfation of tamoxifen metabolites, resulting in their inactivation and clearance [67]. It has been suggested that patients who have reduced SULT1A1 activity would have decreased clearance of 4-OH-TAM and increased treatment efficacy [68]. Comparison of tamoxifen and its metabolites in patients who have the low-activity SULT1A1*2 and the wild-type allele showed no significant differences in the plasma concentrations of tamoxifen metabolites [49]. Some reports have concluded that tamoxifen-treated patients who have the *2 variant have an increased risk for cancer recurrence and death [53,55,68]. However, in a more recent study with 677 tamoxifen-treated postmenopausal women, no association between treatment outcome and the SULT1A1 genotype was found [54,69].

Future directions

In the last 5 to 10 years, much progress has been made regarding not only the relative activity of tamoxifen metabolites but also in understanding the influence of CYP2D6 genotype in response to tamoxifen treatment. The current data strongly suggest that postmenopausal women considering tamoxifen therapy for breast cancer treatment or prevention will greatly benefit from CYP2D6 genotyping. This genotyping should include the most common alleles with null and decreased activity. If possible, in cases where these alleles are present, alternative therapies, such as aromatase inhibitors or raloxifene, should be considered. Unfortunately, most studies have been conducted in postmenopausal women and no published data are available on the benefits of CYP2D6 genotyping and tamoxifen treatment outcomes in premenopausal women, despite tamoxifen being the primary antihormonal therapy for premenopausal patients who have breast cancer. This important area is one that will benefit from additional research and prospective studies. Similarly, thus far, not enough consistent data on a large number of patients exist to support the usefulness of genotyping the other enzymes involved in tamoxifen metabolism. Additional well-controlled clinical studies will aid in clarifying the usefulness of these genetic variants in tamoxifen treatment outcome and whether genotyping for these enzymes should be included in clinical practice.

Summary

The addition of genotypic information to clinical decision making has led to improvements in identifying a subset of patients likely to respond poorly to irinotecan and tamoxifen. However, much remains to be done in terms of optimizing the application of genetic testing to the use of these chemotherapeutics. An important need exists for prospective studies incorporating more comprehensive molecular testing of UGT1A1, CYP2D6, and other related enzymes capable of metabolizing irinotecan and tamoxifen. The amount of genetic analysis required for such an undertaking is overwhelming but is likely essential if the goal is to unravel the contribution of multiple enzymes to patient response. The usefulness of monitoring the levels of irinotecan, tamoxifen, and their metabolites as a complement to enzyme genotype is not currently established, but it may prove essential for predicting outcome in patients who have intermediate-activity genotypes or those treated concomitantly with enzyme inhibitors or inducers. It is commendable that regulatory agencies have taken notice of the ability of pharmacogenetics to predict toxicity or therapeutic failure; however, further refinement of the recommendations for use of irinotecan and tamoxifen will undoubtedly be required as greater understanding of the genetic variables involved unfolds.

References

[1] Package insert for irinotecan as available on the FDA website, http://www.fda.gov/. Available at:Accessed March 3, 2008.

[2] US clinical trials registry, http://clinicaltrials.gov/. Available at:Accessed March 3, 2008.

[3] Wierdl M, Tsurkan L, Hyatt JL, et al. An improved human carboxylesterase for enzyme/prodrug therapy with CPT-11. Cancer Gene Ther 2008;15(3):183–92.

[4] Hanioka N, Ozawa S, Jinno H, et al. Interaction of irinotecan (CPT-11) and its active metabolite 7-ethyl-10-hydroxycamptothecin (SN-38) with human cytochrome P450 enzymes. Drug Metab Dispos 2002;30(4):391–6.

[5] McLeod HL, Watters JW. Irinotecan pharmacogenetics: is it time to intervene? J Clin Oncol 2004;22(8):1356–9.

[6] Ramchandani RP, Wang Y, Booth BP, et al. The role of SN-38 exposure, UGT1A1*28 polymorphism, and baseline bilirubin level in predicting severe irinotecan toxicity. J Clin Pharmacol 2007;47(1):78–86.

[7] Kim TW, Innocenti F. Insights, challenges, and future directions in irinogenetics. Ther Drug Monit 2007;29(3):265–70.

[8] Nagar S, Remmel RP. Uridine diphosphoglucuronosyltransferase pharmacogenetics and cancer. Oncogene 2006;25(11):1659–72.

[9] Innocenti F, Undevia SD, Iyer L, et al. Genetic variants in the UDP-glucuronosyltransferase 1A1 gene predict the risk of severe neutropenia of irinotecan. J Clin Oncol 2004;22(8):1382–8.

[10] Innocenti F, Ratain MJ. Pharmacogenetics of irinotecan: clinical perspectives on the utility of genotyping. Pharmacogenomics 2006;7(8):1211–21.

[11] O'Dwyer PJ, Catalano RB. Uridine diphosphate glucuronosyltransferase (UGT) 1A1 and irinotecan: practical pharmacogenomics arrives in cancer therapy. J Clin Oncol 2006; 24(28):4534–8.

[12] Haga SB, Thummel KE, Burke W. Adding pharmacogenetics information to drug labels: lessons learned. Pharmacogenet Genomics 2006;16(12):847–54.

[13] Ando Y, Fujita K, Sasaki Y, et al. UGT1AI*6 and UGT1A1*27 for individualized irinotecan chemotherapy. Curr Opin Mol Ther 2007;9(3):258–62.

[14] Sai K, Saito Y, Sakamoto H, et al. Importance of UDP-glucuronosyltransferase 1A1(*)6 for irinotecan toxicities in Japanese cancer patients. Cancer Lett 2008;261(2):165–71.

[15] Jinno H, Tanaka-Kagawa T, Hanioka N, et al. Glucuronidation of 7-ethyl-10-hydroxy-camptothecin (SN-38), an active metabolite of irinotecan (CPT-11), by human UGT1A1 variants, G71R, P229Q, and Y486D. Drug Metab Dispos 2003;31(1):108–13.

[16] Gagne JF, Montminy V, Belanger P, et al. Common human UGT1A polymorphisms and the altered metabolism of irinotecan active metabolite 7-ethyl-10-hydroxycamptothecin (SN-38). Mol Pharmacol 2002;62(3):608–17.

[17] Hoskins JM, Goldberg RM, Qu P, et al. UGT1A1*28 genotype and irinotecan-induced neutropenia: dose matters. J Natl Cancer Inst 2007;99(17):1290–5.

[18] Stewart CF, Panetta JC, O'Shaughnessy MA, et al. UGT1A1 promoter genotype correlates with SN-38 pharmacokinetics, but not severe toxicity in patients receiving low-dose irinotecan. J Clin Oncol 2007;25(18):2594–600.

[19] Bomgaars LR, Bernstein M, Krailo M, et al. Phase II trial of irinotecan in children with refractory solid tumors: a Children's Oncology Group Study. J Clin Oncol 2007;25(29): 4622–7.

[20] Rodriguez J, Zarate R, Bandres E, et al. Combining chemotherapy and targeted therapies in metastatic colorectal cancer. World J Gastroenterol 2007;13(44):5867–76.

[21] Cummings J, Ethell BT, Jardine L, et al. Glucuronidation as a mechanism of intrinsic drug resistance in human colon cancer: reversal of resistance by food additives. Cancer Res 2003; 63(23):8443–50.

[22] Innocenti F, Vokes EE, Ratain MJ. Irinogenetics: what is the right star? J Clin Oncol 2006; 24(15):2221–4.

[23] Villeneuve L, Girard H, Fortier LC, et al. Novel functional polymorphisms in the UGT1A7 and UGT1A9 glucuronidating enzymes in Caucasian and African-American subjects and their impact on the metabolism of 7-ethyl-10-hydroxycamptothecin and flavopiridol anticancer drugs. J Pharmacol Exp Ther 2003;307(1):117–28.

[24] Paoluzzi L, Singh AS, Price DK, et al. Influence of genetic variants in UGT1A1 and UGT1A9 on the in vivo glucuronidation of SN-38. J Clin Pharmacol 2004;44(8):854–60.

[25] Ando M, Ando Y, Sekido Y, et al. Genetic polymorphisms of the UDP-glucuronosyltransferase 1A7 gene and irinotecan toxicity in Japanese cancer patients. Jpn J Cancer Res 2002; 93(5):591–7.

[26] Carlini LE, Meropol NJ, Bever J, et al. UGT1A7 and UGT1A9 polymorphisms predict response and toxicity in colorectal cancer patients treated with capecitabine/irinotecan. Clin Cancer Res 2005;11(3):1226–36.

[27] Fujita K, Ando Y, Nagashima F, et al. Genetic linkage of UGT1A7 and UGT1A9 polymorphisms to UGT1A1*6 is associated with reduced activity for SN-38 in Japanese patients with cancer. Cancer Chemother Pharmacol 2007;60(4):515–22.

[28] Baudhuin LM, Highsmith WE, Skierka J, et al. Comparison of three methods for genotyping the UGT1A1 (TA)n repeat polymorphism. Clin Biochem 2007;40(9–10):710–7.

[29] Huang CK, Dulau A, Su-Rick CJ, et al. Validation of rapid polymerase chain reaction-based detection of all length polymorphisms in the UGT 1A1 gene promoter. Diagn Mol Pathol 2007;16(1):50–3.

[30] Araki K, Fujita K, Ando Y, et al. Pharmacogenetic impact of polymorphisms in the coding region of the UGT1A1 gene on SN-38 glucuronidation in Japanese patients with cancer. Cancer Sci 2006;97(11):1255–9.

[31] Ramsay EC, Anantha M, Zastre J, et al. Irinophore C: a liposome formulation of irinotecan with substantially improved therapeutic efficacy against a panel of human xenograft tumors. Clin Cancer Res 2008;14(4):1208–17.

[32] Fisher B, Costantino JP, Wickerham DL, et al. Tamoxifen for prevention of breast cancer: report of the National Surgical Adjuvant Breast and Bowel Project P-1 Study. J Natl Cancer Inst 1998;90(18):1371–88.

[33] Colleoni M, Gelber S, Goldhirsch A, et al. Tamoxifen after adjuvant chemotherapy for pre-menopausal women with lymph node-positive breast cancer: International Breast Cancer Study Group Trial 13-93. J Clin Oncol 2006;24(9):1332–41.

[34] Early Breast Cancer Trialists Collaborative Group. Effects of chemotherapy and hormonal therapy for early breast cancer on recurrence and 15-year survival: an overview of the randomised trials. Lancet 2005;365(9472):1687–717.

[35] Osborne CK. Tamoxifen in the treatment of breast cancer. N Engl J Med 1998;339(22): 1609–18.

[36] Jordan VC, Collins MM, Rowsby L, et al. A monohydroxylated metabolite of tamoxifen with potent antioestrogenic activity. J Endocrinol 1977;75(2):305–16.

[37] Lien EA, Solheim E, Lea OA, et al. Distribution of 4-hydroxy-N-desmethyltamoxifen and other tamoxifen metabolites in human biological fluids during tamoxifen treatment. Cancer Res 1989;49(8):2175–83.

[38] Crewe HK, Notley LM, Wunsch RM, et al. Metabolism of tamoxifen by recombinant human cytochrome P450 enzymes: formation of the 4-hydroxy, 4'-hydroxy and N-desmethyl metabolites and isomerization of trans-4-hydroxytamoxifen. Drug Metab Dispos 2000; 30(8):869–74.

[39] Stearns V, Beebe KL, Iyengar M, et al. Paroxetine controlled release in the treatment of menopausal hot flashes: a randomized controlled trial. JAMA 2003;289(21):2827–34.

[40] Desta Z, Ward BA, Soukhova NV, et al. Comprehensive evaluation of tamoxifen sequential biotransformation by the human cytochrome P450 system in vitro: prominent roles for CYP3A and CYP2D6. J Pharmacol Exp Ther 2004;310(3):1062–75.

[41] Coller JK, Krebsfaenger N, Klein K, et al. The influence of CYP2B6, CYP2C9 and CYP2D6 genotypes on the formation of the potent antioestrogen Z-4-hydroxy-tamoxifen in human liver. Br J Clin Pharmacol 2002;54(2):157–67.

[42] Borgna JL, Rochefort H. Hydroxylated metabolites of tamoxifen are formed in vivo and bound to estrogen receptor in target tissues. J Biolumin Chemilumin 1981;256(2): 859–68.

[43] Robertson DW, Katzenellenbogen JA, Long DJ, et al. Tamoxifen antiestrogens. A comparison of the activity, pharmacokinetics, and metabolic activation of the cis and trans isomers of tamoxifen. J Steroid Biochem 1982;16(1):1–13.

[44] Coezy E, Borgna JL, Rochefort H. Tamoxifen and metabolites in MCF7 cells: correlation between binding to estrogen receptor and inhibition of cell growth. Cancer Res 1982; 42(1):317–23.

[45] Johnson MD, Zuo H, Lee KH, et al. Pharmacological characterization of 4-hydroxy-N-desmethyl tamoxifen, a novel active metabolite of tamoxifen. Breast Cancer Res Treat 2004; 85(2):151–9.

[46] Lim YC, Desta Z, Flockhart DA, et al. Endoxifen (4-hydroxy-N-desmethyl-tamoxifen) has anti-estrogenic effects in breast cancer cells with potency similar to 4-hydroxy-tamoxifen. Cancer Chemother Pharmacol 2005;55(5):471–8.

[47] Wilkinson GR. Drug metabolism and variability among patients in drug response. N Engl J Med 2005;352(21):2211–21.

[48] Ingelman-Sundberg M, Sim SC, Gomez A, et al. Influence of cytochrome P450 polymorphisms on drug therapies: pharmacogenetic, pharmacoepigenetic and clinical aspects. Pharmacol Ther 2007;116(3):496–526.

[49] Jin Y, Desta Z, Stearns V, et al. CYP2D6 genotype, antidepressant use, and tamoxifen metabolism during adjuvant breast cancer treatment. J Natl Cancer Inst 2005;97(1):30–9.

[50] Borges S, Desta Z, Li L, et al. Quantitative effect of CYP2D6 genotype and inhibitors on tamoxifen metabolism: implication for optimization of breast cancer treatment. Clin Pharmacol Ther 2006;80(1):61–74.

[51] Goetz MP, Rae JM, Suman VJ, et al. Pharmacogenetics of tamoxifen biotransformation is associated with clinical outcomes of efficacy and hot flashes. J Clin Oncol 2005;23(36): 9312–8.

[52] Bonanni B, Macis D, Maisonneuve P, et al. Polymorphism in the CYP2D6 tamoxifen-metabolizing gene influences clinical effect but not hot flashes: data from the Italian Tamoxifen Trial. J Clin Oncol 2006;24(22):3708–9, [author reply: 3709].

[53] Nowell SA, Ahn J, Rae JM, et al. Association of genetic variation in tamoxifen-metabolizing enzymes with overall survival and recurrence of disease in breast cancer patients. Breast Cancer Res Treat 2005;91(3):249–58.

[54] Wegman P, Elingarami S, Carstensen J, et al. Genetic variants of CYP3A5, CYP2D6, SULT1A1, UGT2B15 and tamoxifen response in postmenopausal patients with breast cancer. Breast Cancer Res 2007;9(1):R7.

[55] Wegman P, Vainikka L, Stal O, et al. Genotype of metabolic enzymes and the benefit of tamoxifen in postmenopausal breast cancer patients. Breast Cancer Res 2005;7(3): R284–90.

[56] Goetz MP, Kamal A, Ames MM. Tamoxifen pharmacogenomics: the role of CYP2D6 as a predictor of drug response. Clin Pharmacol Ther 2008;83(1):160–6.

[57] Goetz MP, Knox SK, Suman VJ, et al. The impact of cytochrome P450 2D6 metabolism in women receiving adjuvant tamoxifen. Breast Cancer Res Treat 2007;101(1):113–21.

[58] Loibl S, Schwedler K, von Minckwitz G, et al. Venlafaxine is superior to clonidine as treatment of hot flashes in breast cancer patients – a double-blind, randomized study. Ann Oncol 2007;18(4):689–93.

[59] Young D. Genetics examined in tamoxifen's effectiveness: recurrence warning urged for labeling. Am J Health Syst Pharm 2006;63(23):2286–96.

[60] Howell A, Cuzick J, Baum M, et al. Results of the ATAC (Arimidex, Tamoxifen, alone or in combination) trial after completion of 5 years' adjuvant treatment for breast cancer. Lancet 2005;365(9453):60–2.

[61] Bevers TB. Raloxifene and the prevention of breast cancer. Expert Opin Pharmacother 2006; 7(16):2301–7.

[62] Vogel VG, Costantino JP, Wickerham DL, et al. Effects of tamoxifen vs raloxifene on the risk of developing invasive breast cancer and other disease outcomes: the NSABP study of tamoxifen and raloxifene (STAR) P-2 trial. JAMA 2006;295(23):2727–41.

[63] Tucker AN, Tkaczuk KA, Lewis LM, et al. Polymorphisms in cytochrome P4503A5 (CYP3A5) may be associated with race and tumor characteristics, but not metabolism and side effects of tamoxifen in breast cancer patients. Cancer Lett 2005;217(1):61–72.

[64] Koch I, Weil R, Wolbold R, et al. Interindividual variability and tissue-specificity in the expression of cytochrome P450 3A mRNA. Drug Metab Dispos 2002;30(10):1108–14.

[65] Westlind-Johnsson A, Malmebo S, Johansson A, et al. Comparative analysis of CYP3A expression in human liver suggests only a minor role for CYP3A5 in drug metabolism. Drug Metab Dispos 2003;31(6):755–61.

[66] Schroth W, Antoniadou L, Fritz P, et al. Breast cancer treatment outcome with adjuvant tamoxifen relative to patient CYP2D6 and CYP2C19 genotypes. J Clin Oncol 2007; 25(33):5187–93.

[67] Chen G, Yin S, Maiti S, et al. 4-Hydroxytamoxifen sulfation metabolism. J Biochem Mol Toxicol 2002;16(6):279–85.

[68] Nowell S, Sweeney C, Winters M, et al. Association between sulfotransferase 1A1 genotype and survival of breast cancer patients receiving tamoxifen therapy. J Natl Cancer Inst 2002; 94(21):1635–40.

[69] Gjerde J, Hauglid M, Breilid H, et al. Effects of CYP2D6 and SULT1A1 genotypes including SULT1A1 gene copy number on tamoxifen metabolism. Ann Oncol 2008;19(1):56–61.

CLINICS IN
LABORATORY
MEDICINE

ELSEVIER
SAUNDERS

Clin Lab Med 28 (2008) 569–579

Pharmacogenetics in Pain Management: the Clinical Need

Lynn R. Webster, MD

*Lifetree Clinical Research and Pain Clinic, 3838 South, 700 East,
Suite 200, Salt Lake City, UT 84106, USA*

Pharmacogenetic therapy in pain patients requires consideration of two different genetic substrates to determine the outcome of pharmacotherapy. The first is the genetic contribution of a variety of different pain types and the second is the genetic influence on drug effectiveness and safety. This article presents evidence of a genetic influence on the prevalence and processing of pain, a discussion of the genetics of drug therapy, and a clinical scenario to illustrate the need to integrate the genetics of pain and pharmacogenetics to achieve the best outcomes.

Genetics of pain

When it comes to nociceptive sensitivity, the stimulus intensity makes a difference and so does the person's experience of pain. Studies to isolate the genetic risk of inheriting a specific pain condition are plentiful, but scientists are only beginning to examine genetic variations that may influence pain processing. If a genetic basis underlies how pain is expressed, including the varying mechanisms of nociceptive, neuropathic, and visceral pain, then the potential exists for new analgesic targets. In the future, the right drug may depend on the patient's genotype.

Financial Disclosures: Advanced Bionic, research-consultant; Alpharma Pharmaceuticals and Ameritox, research; Aztra Zenca, research; Cephalon, consultant; CoMentis, research; Covidien, consultant; Durect, research; Elan, research-consultant; Elite, research; Forest, research; GlaxoSmithKline, research; Jazz, research; King Pharmaceutical, research-consultant; LLC, research-consultant; Medtronic, research-consultant; Merck, research; Nektar, research; Nervo, consultant; NeurogesX, research; Pfizer, research; Pain Therapeutics, Inc., research; Purdue, research; QRx, research; Respironics, research; Takeda, research; Torreypines, research; Zars, research.

E-mail address: lynnw@lifetreepain.com

doi:10.1016/j.cll.2008.05.005   *labmed.theclinics.com*

Pain expression is also influenced by environmental factors, such as cultural attitudes, attention, and stress. Fibromyalgia (FM), tension headaches, and irritable bowel syndrome are a few of the functional pain conditions influenced by environmental factors. Environment may sometimes confound efforts to isolate genetic contributions in clinical studies, and these effects should be kept in mind.

Candidate gene studies in pain

The clinical needs in pain management are driven by a broad spectrum of pain sensitivity observed in patients. Clinical observation suggests large interindividual differences in pain sensitivity (Fig. 1), and research confirms that view [1]. Examples of pain conditions that persist in a minority of patients include diabetes with diabetic peripheral neuropathy, herpes zoster with postherpetic neuralgia, lumbar disc degeneration with low back pain, and whiplash injuries with cervicalgia [2]. Some of the variance is explained by age, severity of stimulus, and environmental factors, but not all. A genetic influence is suggested by results showing that inbred mouse strains respond differently to the same acute and chronic pain stimuli [3–5].

Allele-based association studies are expected to shed light on the mystery of why pain persists in some patients but not others after nearly identical tissue damage. At present, close to 200 candidate genes have been identified that may be involved in pain processing [2], and there may be thousands more. The 200 molecules have been categorized by their frequency of occurrence in chronic neuropathic pain conditions and further by the strength of evidence, frequency of the specific variant, and likelihood that a genetic polymorphism[1] alters function (Table 1).

Separating genetic from environmental factors is usually best explored through twin studies. Patients with migraine [6–8], back pain [9], and menstrual pain [10] have been studied in twins with estimates of genetic contribution to pain-related traits reported as 39% to 58%, 50%, and 55%, respectively. The following subsections further elucidate findings related to genetics in specific pain conditions.

Low back pain

Low back pain is the leading cause of job-related disability in the United States and second only to headache as the most common neurologic complaint [11]. The causes are many, but degeneration of the spine and intervertebral discs are frequently blamed. Conventional scientific consensus says intervertebral disc degeneration and other spinal abnormalities are largely mechanical, but recent evidence has implicated genetic and biochemical

---

[1] A polymorphism is a variation in DNA sequencing that occurs in greater than 1% of the population; in contrast, a mutation occurs in less than 1 % (Stamer UM, Stüber F. The pharmacogenetics of analgesia. Expert Opin Pharmacother 2007;8(14):2235–45).

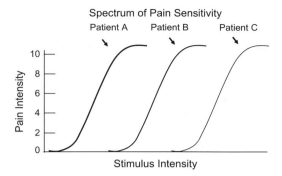

Fig. 1. A simulation of interindividual variability in pain sensitivity: Patient A has increased sensitivity, Patient B has a normal response, and patient C has decreased sensitivity.

mechanisms. In a study of 804 Chinese volunteers, age 18 to 55, investigators found that a polymorphism—the Trp2 allele COL9A2 coding for alpha2 chain of collagen IX—is associated with a fourfold increase in the risk of developing annular tears in people ages 30 to 39 years. The molecule was associated with a 2.4-fold increase in the risk of developing degenerative disc disease and end-plate herniations in people ages 40 to 49 years [12]. In addition, the presence of Trp2 predicted the severity of disc degeneration. The effect was more apparent in some age groups than in others. Boosting evidence that genetic risk factors vary among ethnicities, the Trp3 allele— shown to increase the risk of lumbar disc disease threefold in Finnish patients [13]—was absent in the Chinese population.

Migraine

Migraine is more prevalent in females (17.1%) than in males (5.6%), and evidence points to an X-chromosome link, specifically at the locus of chromosome Xq24-28 [14,15]. High anxiety and certain types of migraines have shown an association with the short (s) allele of the serotonin transporter gene 5HTTLPR polymorphism [16]. Furthermore, hemiplegic migraine is associated with a gene on the 19p13 chromosome, presenting evidence that different types of migraines may be linked to different genetic polymorphisms [17].

Fibromyalgia

Fibromyalgia is a disease characterized by diffuse musculoskeletal pain and generalized tender points. It affects approximately 2% of the general population, and women are more susceptible than men [18]. Studies show FM to be more prevalent within families than in the general population [19,20]; however, the problem of isolating environmental and genetic factors continues. Some evidence exists that FM is autosomal dominant [21]. An

Table 1
High-priority candidate genes for human neuropathic pain

Gene	Molecule	Variant	Location
IL6	Interleukin 6	G 174 C	Promoter
NOS1	Neuronal nitric oxide synthase	AAT VNTR	Intron 20
IL1B	Interleukin 1β	C 511 T	Promoter
TNF α	Tumor necrosis factor α	G 308 A	Promoter
SLC6A4	Serotonin transporter	5HTTLPR	Promoter
GDNF	Glial-derived nerve factor	(AGG) (n)	3' UTR
BDKRB2	Bradykinin receptor 2	C 58 T	Promoter
COMT	Catechol-O-methyltransferase	Val 158 Met	Exon 3
NOS2A	Inducible nitric oxide synthase	CCTTTn repeat	Promoter
PDYN	Prodynorphin	68 bp repeat	Promoter
OPRM1	μ-opioid receptor	Asn 40 Asp	Exon 1
IL10	Interleukin 10	A 1082 G	Promoter
BDKRB1	Bradykinin receptor 1	G 699 T	Promoter
TH	Tyrosine hydroxylase	Val 81 Met	Exon 3
RET	Protooncogene (tyrosine kinase)	Gly 691 Ser	Exon 11
GRIK3	Kainate (glutamate) receptor	Ser 310 Ala	Coding
IL13	Interleukin 13	Arg 130 Gln	Coding
BDNF	Brain-derived nerve factor	Val 66 Met	Exon 5
ADRA2A	α_{2A}-Adrenergic receptor	C 1291 G	Promoter
CACNA2D2	Calcium channel subunit	G 845 C	Intron 2

Data from Belfer I, Wu T, Kingman A, et al. Candidate gene studies of human pain mechanisms: methods for optimizing choice of polymorphisms and sample size. Anesthesiology 2004;100(6):1562–72.

association of a gene for FM with human leukocyte antigen has been reported [22] and further supported by research conducted in 40 multicase families with FM [23]. The T102C polymorphism of the 5-HT2A serotonin receptor gene may contribute to nociception in FM, though a link has not been established in FM etiology. An investigation of the T102C allele found that FM patients exhibited a decrease in T/T and an increase in T/C and C/C genotypes when compared with healthy controls [24]. The pain scores for the T/T genotype were significantly higher then for T/C or C/C polymorphisms.

Several disorders associated with fibromyalgia have similar symptoms and also appear to have a similar neuropathology. A large population-based study using the Swedish Twin Registry determined that genetic factors contribute to the co-occurrence of FM with psychiatric disorders, including major depression, generalized anxiety disorder, and eating disorders [25]. Significant co-occurrences were found between FM and chronic fatigue, joint pain, depressive symptoms, and irritable bowel syndrome. Collectively termed "functional somatic syndromes," these conditions share many clinical features, which point to a shared mechanism for pain sensitivity.

A role has been suggested for polymorphisms of genes in the serotoninergic, dopaminergic, and catecholaminergic systems, which are associated with FM and additional comorbid conditions [26]. The polymorphisms could result in an imbalance of many neurochemicals, leading to the somatic complaints and depression common in FM and related disorders.

Hereditary disorders insensitive to pain

A confirmation of the genetic association to perceived pain is found in the five congenital disorders characterized by defects in normal sensation that have been documented to date (Box 1, [27–31]). Understanding genomic involvement with pain may lead to more precise pain therapies.

Genetics of analgesia

Clinicians who treat pain have always known that the response to opioids varies widely among patients. Differences in bioavailability and pain stimuli explain some of this difference, but genetic makeup is likely a strong factor. Clinicians struggle with finding a consistent response to pain medications because of this tremendous interpatient response. There are several ways genetics influence drug response: through drug metabolism enzymes, drug transporters, opioid or other pain medication receptors, or structures involved in the perception and processing of pain.

Pharmacogenetics describes the effects of polymorphic genes on the enzymes that metabolize drugs. It has been shown that a variation in amino acid sequence replacing an arginine and a serine by a histidine (R265H) and a proline (S268P) residue, respectively, at the mu opioid receptor can change receptor signaling after stimulation with morphine [32]. Ethnic groups are known to vary in response to opioid medications. Caucasians are more prone to sedation and respiratory depression than Asians are, and Native Americans display even more depression of the ventilatory response than do Caucasians [33,34]. Animal studies provide further ballast: in one study, inbred laboratory mice (CXBK) showed no response to levels of morphine that are analgesic for more than 90% of typical mice [35].

What follows is a consideration of research involving certain genetic polymorphisms and their association with increased or reduced drug sensitivity. The evidence, so far, implicates only a few genes in pain processing.

Box 1. Congenital disorders characterized by defects in normal pain processing

Congenital insensitivity to pain with anhidrosis [27]
Familial dysautonomia (also called Riley-Day syndrome
   or HSAN III) [28]
Lesch-Nyhan syndrome [29]
Tourette's syndrome [30]
De Lange syndrome [31]

Cytochrome P450 2D6 gene

Among the most studied factors in drug metabolism is the CYP2D6, one of the cytochrome P450 enzymes, which are a super-family of drug-metabolizing enzymes that have shown variations in large populations [36]. Researchers have described more than 75 CYP2D6 alleles [36], and further study has found that patients who rapidly metabolize therapeutic drugs have multiple copies of the CYP2D6 gene [37]. Polymorphism of this gene helps explain tremendous individual differences in opioid requirements.

Here, too, research has uncovered notable differences in the frequencies of alleles among different nations and ethnic groups: close to 29% of people in parts of East Africa may have multiple copies of CYP2D6, while the pattern is rare in Northern Europeans [38]. In fact, CYP2D6 gene duplication has been shown to occur in less than 2.6% of Caucasians [39].

OPRM1 118G

The mu-opioid receptor encoded by genetic locus OPRM1 is a prime site of action for endogenous opioid peptides and, thus, of interest to genetic investigators. Laboratory and clinical evidence has shown increased opioid requirements in patients with the OPRM1 118G polymorphism [40–42]. Of 120 patients who underwent total knee arthroplasty, patients who were 118G homozygotes consumed significantly more morphine than did patients who were 118A homozygotes or heterozygotes [41]. A further study found significantly greater opioid consumption to achieve pain control in 118G homozygotes compared with 118A homozygotes for hysterectomy patients during the first 24 hours postsurgery [42].

Catechol-O-methyltransferase gene

Catechol-O-methyltransferase metabolizes catecholamines and is important for dopaminergic and adrenergic/noradrenergic neurotransmission. A common polymorphism at amino acid position 158 (Val158Met) has been shown to impact human pain response [43]. Individuals with a homozygous methionine-158 genotype showed diminished regional mu-opioid system response to pain when compared with heterozygotes, and also demonstrated higher sensory and affective ratings of pain. Cancer patients with the Met/Met genotype also have shown a heightened need for morphine [44]. However, other research has found only a weak association between polymorphisms in the monoamine neurotransmitter systems and postsurgical pain response [45].

Melanocortin-1 receptor gene

The Melanocortin-1 receptor (MC1R) gene variants offer additional interesting evidence of the potential for highly targeted analgesia based on sex and other differences. There is evidence that women, more than men, respond to kappa-induced analgesia [46], which is mediated by the MC1R [47]. Women carrying two nonfunctional alleles displayed greater pentazocine (kappa agonist) analgesic response compared with women with one or no such alleles, or men [48]. Furthermore, 75% of individuals with red hair and pale skin phenotypes carry two or more inactivating variants of the MC1R [48].

Affect of genotype variants on dose

The opioid dose required for analgesia will be affected by genotype variants. One dose does not fit all. For example, a patient with the variant of OPRM1 may require twice the standard morphine dose to be effective. This variability in clinical effect among patients based on genotype emphasizes the need to perform pharmacogenetic assessments in patients, perhaps leading to the concept of "pharmacogenetic-based dose adaptation" [49].

Joining the genetics of pain and analgesia for clinical utility

Pharmacotherapy for chronic pain will encompass the genetic research on the variability of pain expression and the variations in response to analgesic medications. One clinical scenario that presents difficulty in this regard lies in initiating doses of methadone for pain.

Initiating methadone: a clinical scenario

Unintentional overdose deaths involving methadone are rising. A report by the National Drug Intelligence Center found methadone deaths rose 390% from 1999 through 2004, a higher rate than for any other opioid [50]. A common scenario in these deaths is accumulation of methadone to a toxic level during initiation for pain therapy or addiction treatment because of an overestimation of tolerance and lack of consideration for methadone's long, variable half-life, according to the United States Substance Abuse and Mental Health Services Administration [51]. Because many deaths from methadone occur within the first few weeks of initiating therapy, poor methadone metabolism in a subset of patients may well be a factor.

The cytochrome P450 (CYP) enzyme system is a key player in methadone metabolism, and research is aimed at discovering which isoenzymes have the most influence. Although its metabolism is complex and research is incomplete, methadone appears to be metabolized mainly by CYP2B6 [52–54]. Testing for this isoenzyme may help identify who is at risk for slow metabolism and, therefore, toxicity from drug accumulation.

The spectrum of medication response

Genotyping for CYP2D6 has resulted in classifying morphine recipients as poor metabolizers, extensive metabolizers, intermediate metabolizers, or ultrarapid metabolizers [55] with consequences for pain sensitivity and opioid consumption. The categorization suggests a spectrum of possible responses from analgesia to lack of efficacy to toxicity after the same doses.

Furthermore, poor metabolism of opioids could compromise the interpretations of urine drug testing administered to ensure compliance with opioid therapy. If genotyping were to reveal poor or ultrarapid opioid metabolizers, clinicians may find quantitative urine drug testing useful in assessing whether patients are consuming their prescriptions as directed or possibly diverting some of them.

Adverse drug reactions

Genetic variations that impact a patient's drug sensitivity can lead to adverse reactions, toxicity, or therapeutic failure [56]. Of 27 drugs frequently cited in adverse drug reaction studies, 59% are metabolized by at least one enzyme with a variant allele known to cause poor metabolism [57]. That compares with 7% to 22% of randomly selected drugs. Tailoring therapy based upon each individual's genotype should yield increased therapeutic effectiveness and minimize adverse effects.

Summary

Each person carries his or her own genetic imprint for pain response and medication sensitivity. How this genetic profile is expressed may be significantly influenced by the environment. Studies of genetic polymorphisms linked to pain syndromes and medication metabolism promise a fresh therapeutic approach where targeted analgesia with fewer side effects may be possible based on genotype.

Acknowledgments

The author would like to thank Beth Dove of Lifetree Clinical Research and Pain Clinic for providing technical writing and manuscript review.

References

[1] Mogil JS. The genetic mediation of individual differences in sensitivity to pain and its inhibition. Proc Natl Acad Sci U S A 1999;96(14):7744–51 [review].
[2] Belfer I, Wu T, Kingman A, et al. Candidate gene studies of human pain mechanisms: methods for optimizing choice of polymorphisms and sample size. Anesthesiology 2004; 100(6):1562–72.
[3] Mogil JS, Wilson SG, Bon K, et al. Heritability of nociception I: responses of 11 inbred mouse strains on 12 measures of nociception. Pain 1999;80(1–2):67–82.
[4] Lariviere WR, Wilson SG, Laughlin TM, et al. Heritability of nociception. III. Genetic relationships among commonly used assays of nociception and hypersensitivity. Pain 2002;97(1–2):75–86.

[5] Seltzer Z, Wu T, Max MB, et al. Mapping a gene for neuropathic pain-related behavior following peripheral neurectomy in the mouse. Pain 2001;93(2):101–6.

[6] Honkasalo ML, Kaprio J, Winter T, et al. Migraine and concomitant symptoms among 8167 adult twin pairs. Headache 1995;35(2):70–8.

[7] Larsson B, Bille B, Pedersen NL. Genetic influence in headaches: a Swedish twin study. Headache 1995;35(9):513–9.

[8] Ziegler DK, Hur YM, Bouchard TJ Jr, et al. Migraine in twins raised together and apart. Headache 1998;38(6):417–22.

[9] Bengtsson B, Thorson J. Back pain: a study of twins. Acta Genet Med Gemellol (Roma) 1991;40(1):83–90.

[10] Treloar SA, Martin NG, Heath AC. Longitudinal genetic analysis of menstrual flow, pain, and limitation in a sample of Australian twins. Behav Genet 1998;28(2):107–16.

[11] National Institute of Neurological Disorders and Stroke. 2003 Low back pain fact sheet. Office of Communications and Public Liaison. National Institutes of Health. Bethesda (MD): NIH Publication No. 03-5161; Available at: http://www.ninds.nih.gov/disorders/backpain/detail_backpain.htm. Updated January 10, 2008. Last accessed March 6, 2008.

[12] Jim JJ, Noponen-Hietala N, Cheung KM, et al. The TRP2 allele of COL9A2 is an age-dependent risk factor for the development and severity of intervertebral disc degeneration. Spine 2005;30(24):2735–42.

[13] Paassilta P, Lohiniva J, Göring HH, et al. Identification of a novel common genetic risk factor for lumbar disk disease. JAMA 2001;285(14):1843–9.

[14] Lipton RB, Bigal ME, Diamond M, et al. Migraine prevalence, disease burden, and the need for preventive therapy. Neurology 2007;68(5):343–9.

[15] Nyholt DR, Curtain RP, Griffiths LR. Familial typical migraine: significant linkage and localization of a gene to Xq24-28. Hum Genet 2000;107(1):18–23.

[16] Gonda X, Rihmer Z, Juhasz G, et al. High anxiety and migraine are associated with the s allele of the 5HTTLPR gene polymorphism. Psychiatry Res 2007;149(1–3):261–6.

[17] Joutel A, Bousser MG, Biousse V, et al. A gene for familial hemiplegic migraine maps to chromosome 19. Nat Genet 1993;5(1):40–5.

[18] Chakrabarty S, Zoorob R. Fibromyalgia. Am Fam Physician 2007;76(2):247–54.

[19] Arnold LM, Hudson JI, Hess EV, et al. Family study of fibromyalgia. Arthritis Rheum 2004; 50(3):944–52.

[20] Buskila D, Neumann L, Hazanov I, et al. Familial aggregation in the fibromyalgia syndrome. Semin Arthritis Rheum 1996;26(3):605–11.

[21] Pellegrino MJ, Waylonis GW, Sommer A. Familial occurrence of primary fibromyalgia. Arch Phys Med Rehabil 1989;70(1):61–3.

[22] Burda CD, Cox FR, Osborne P. Histocompatability antigens in the fibrositis (fibromyalgia) syndrome. Clin Exp Rheumatol 1986;4(4):355–8.

[23] Yunus MB, Khan MA, Rawlings KK, et al. Genetic linkage analysis of multicase families with fibromyalgia syndrome. J Rheumatol 1999;26(2):408–12.

[24] Bondy B, Spaeth M, Offenbaecher M, et al. The T102C polymorphism of the 5-HT2A-receptor gene in fibromyalgia. Neurobiol Dis 1999;6(5):433–9.

[25] Kato K, Sullivan P, Evengård B, et al. Chronic widespread pain and its comorbidities: a population-based study. Arch Intern Med 2006;166(15):1649–54.

[26] Buskila D, Sarzi-Puttini P, Ablin JN. The genetics of fibromyalgia syndrome. Pharmacogenomics 2007;8(1):67–74.

[27] Berkovitch M, Copeliovitch L, Tauber T, et al. Hereditary insensitivity to pain with anhidrosis. Pediatr Neurol 1998;19(3):227–9.

[28] Blumenfeld A, Slaugenhaupt SA, Axelrod FB, et al. Localization of the gene for familial dysautonomia on chromosome 9 and definition of DNA markers for genetic diagnosis. Nat Genet 1993;4(2):160–4.

[29] Shapira J, Zilberman Y, Becker A. Lesch-Nyhan syndrome: a nonextracting approach to prevent mutilation. Spec Care Dentist 1985;5(5):210–2.

[30] Lowe O. Tourette's syndrome: management of oral complications. ASDC J Dent Child 1986;53(6):456–60.

[31] Shear CS, Nyhan WL, Kirman BH, et al. Self-mutilative behavior as a feature of the de Lange syndrome. J Pediatr 1971;78(3):506–9.

[32] Befort K, Filiol D, Decalliot FM, et al. A single nucleotide polymorphic mutation in the human μ-opioid receptor severely impairs receptor signaling. J Biol Chem 2001;276:3130–7.

[33] Zhou HH, Sheller JR, Nu HE, et al. Ethnic differences in response to morphine. Clin Pharmacol Ther 1993;54:507–13.

[34] Cepeda MS, Farrar JT, Roa JH, et al. Ethnicity influences morphine pharmacokinetics and pharmacodynamics. Clin Pharmacol Ther 2001;70(4):351–61.

[35] Schuller AG, King MA, Zhang J, et al. Retention of heroin and morphine-6 beta-glucuronide analgesia in a new line of mice lacking exon 1 of MOR-1. Nat Neurosci 1999;2(2):151–6.

[36] Weinshilboum R. Inheritance and drug response. N Engl J Med 2003;348(6):529–37.

[37] Johansson I, Lundqvist E, Bertilsson L, et al. Inherited amplification of an active gene in the cytochrome P450 CYP2D locus as a cause of ultrarapid metabolism of debrisoquine. Proc Natl Acad Sci U S A 1993;90:11825–9.

[38] Aklillu E, Persson I, Bertilsson L, et al. Frequent distribution of ultrarapid metabolizers of debrisoquine in an Ethiopian population carrying duplicated and multiduplicated functional CYP2D6 alleles. J Pharmacol Exp Ther 1996;278:441–6.

[39] Sachse C, Brockmöller J, Bauer S, et al. Cytochrome P450 2D6 variants in a Caucasian population: allele frequencies and phenotypic consequences. Am J Hum Genet 1997;60(2):284–95.

[40] Klepstad P, Rakvåg TT, Kaasa S, et al. The 118 A > G polymorphism in the human mu-opioid receptor gene may increase morphine requirements in patients with pain caused by malignant disease. Acta Anaesthesiol Scand 2004;48(10):1232–9.

[41] Chou WY, Yang LC, Lu HF, et al. Association of mu-opioid receptor gene polymorphism (A118G) with variations in morphine consumption for analgesia after total knee arthroplasty. Acta Anaesthesiol Scand 2006;50(7):787–92.

[42] Chou WY, Wang CH, Liu PH, et al. Human opioid receptor A118G polymorphism affects intravenous patient-controlled analgesia morphine consumption after total abdominal hysterectomy. Anesthesiology 2006;105(2):334–7.

[43] Zubieta JK, Heitzeg MM, Smith YR, et al. COMT val158met genotype affects mu-opioid neurotransmitter responses to a pain stressor. Science 2003;299(5610):1240–3.

[44] Rakvåg TT, Klepstad P, Baar C, et al. The Val158Met polymorphism of the human catechol-O-methyltransferase (COMT) gene may influence morphine requirements in cancer pain patients. Pain 2005;116(1–2):73–8.

[45] Kim H, Lee H, Rowan J, et al. Genetic polymorphisms in monoamine neurotransmitter systems show only weak association with acute post-surgical pain in humans. Mol Pain 2006;2:24.

[46] Gear RW, Miaskowski C, Gordon NC, et al. Kappa-opioids produce significantly greater analgesia in women than in men. Nat Med 1996;2(11):1248–50.

[47] Mogil JS, Wilson SG, Chesler EJ, et al. The melanocortin-1 receptor gene mediates female-specific mechanisms of analgesia in mice and humans. Proc Natl Acad Sci U S A 2003;100(8):4867–72.

[48] Mogil JS, Ritchie J, Smith SB, et al. Melanocortin-1 receptor gene variants affect pain and mu-opioid analgesia in mice and humans. J Med Genet 2005;42(7):583–7.

[49] Lötsch J, Geisslinger G. Current evidence for a genetic modulation of the response to analgesics. Pain 2006;121(1–2):1–5.

[50] Methadone diversion, abuse, and misuse: deaths increasing at alarming rate Product No. 2007-Q0317-001. Johnstown, PA: US Department of Justice, National Drug Intelligence Center; 2007.

[51] Center for Substance Abuse Treatment. Methadone-associated mortality: report of a national assessment, May 8–9, 2003. Rockville (MD): CSAT Publication No. 28-03; Center for Substance Abuse Treatment, Substance Abuse and Mental Health Services Administration. 2004.

[52] Clark JD. Understanding methadone metabolism: a foundation for safer use. Anesthesiology 2008;108(3):351–2.
[53] Totah RA, Sheffels P, Roberts T, et al. Role of CYP2B6 in stereoselective human methadone metabolism. Anesthesiology 2008;108(3):363–74.
[54] Crettol S, Déglon JJ, Besson J, et al. ABCB1 and cytochrome P450 genotypes and phenotypes: influence on methadone plasma levels and response to treatment. Clin Pharmacol Ther 2006;80(6):668–81.
[55] Candiotti KA, Yang Z, Curia L, et al. The impact of CYP2D6 genetic polymorphism on postoperative morphine consumption. Presented at the 24th Annual Meeting of the American Academy of Pain Medicine. Orlando (FL) (February 12–16, 2008). [Poster 120].
[56] Stamer UM, Stüber F. The pharmacogenetics of analgesia. Expert Opin Pharmacother 2007; 8(14):2235–45 [review].
[57] Phillips KA, Veenstra DL, Oren E, et al. Potential role of pharmacogenomics in reducing adverse drug reactions: a systematic review. JAMA 2001;286(18):2270–9.

ELSEVIER
SAUNDERS

CLINICS IN
LABORATORY
MEDICINE

Clin Lab Med 28 (2008) 581–598

The Value of CYP2D6 and OPRM1 Pharmacogenetic Testing for Opioid Therapy

Kristen K. Reynolds, PhD[a,b],*,
Bronwyn Ramey-Hartung, PhD[a],
Saeed A. Jortani, PhD[a,b]

[a]*PG$_{XL}$ Laboratories, 201 E. Jefferson Street, Suite 309, Louisville, KY 40202, USA*
[b]*Department of Pathology and Laboratory Medicine, University of Louisville
School of Medicine, Louisville, KY 40292, USA*

More than 80 million people in the United States suffer annually from serious pain, the vast majority, roughly 85%, suffering from chronic manifestations such as lower back pain, arthritis, and headache [1,2]. The costs associated with pain management are estimated to be over $61 billion annually, primarily because of lost productivity at work [3]. Thus, satisfactory treatment of pain is paramount for patients to return to a productive lifestyle.

In managing pain, clinicians and their patients often face decisions that involve choosing the most appropriate pharmacologic agent, to contemplating nonpharmacologic modalities. If the choice is drug therapy for relieving pain (ie, analgesics), nonsteroidal anti-inflammatory drugs (NSAIDs) and opioids are the primary choices. Additional drug types such as the antidepressants and anti-epileptics have also been used to treat neurologic pain. More than 20 years ago, the World Health Organization (WHO) recommended a stepwise and "ladder" approach to management of pain [4]. Administration of non-opioid medications (adjuvants) is considered for mild pain as an initial step. For moderate pain, mild opioids such as codeine, with or without the adjuvants, and non-opioids are considered next. For persistent moderate to severe pain, strong opioids such as morphine, with or without adjuvants, and non-opioids are considered [5]. The effectiveness of this approach has been questioned and studied over the past several years [6].

* Corresponding author. PG$_{XL}$ Laboratories, 201 E. Jefferson Street, Suite 309, Louisville, KY 40202, USA
E-mail address: kreynolds@pgxlab.com (K.K. Reynolds).

Regardless, the popularity of the WHO analgesic ladder in various fields of medicine is evident [7].

Pain management medications

Nonsteroidal Anti-Inflammatory Drugs

NSAIDs are primarily considered in the management of mild to moderate nociceptive pain. They are particularly useful for inflammatory states and pain involving the musculoskeletal system [8]. Several members of this class may cause gastric disturbances, gastrointestinal (GI) bleeding, platelet aggregation inhibition, and nephrotoxicity. Blockade of cyclooxygenase-2 (COX-2) has been a relatively recent alternative to produce analgesia and anti-inflammatory effects without the GI or bleeding side effects; however, COX-2 inhibitors are relatively expensive while being generally equipotent to other NSAIDs. In situations where NSAIDs are required and the risk of GI or bleeding side effects cannot be tolerated, COX-2 inhibitors are considered as great alternatives [9]. Despite these advantages, COX-2 inhibitors increase the risk of myocardial infarction and stroke [10].

Opioids

Opioids are a group of narcotic drugs capable of relieving pain, but that can induce sleep, become addictive, and cause stupor, coma, or death in higher doses. There are two major classes of alkaloids in the poppy plant (*Papaver somniferum*) referred to as isoquinolines and phenanthrenes. Morphine, codeine, and thebaine are the major phenanthrenes with binding affinity to the opioid receptors. The term opiate refers to the naturally occurring analogs in the poppy plant as well as their semisynthetic congeners [11]. The word opioid is a broader term and refers to semisynthetic or synthetic substances derived from or resembling the alkaloids in the poppy plant as well as the endogenous neurotransmitters with affinity for the opioid receptors (described in a later section). An alternative definition for opioid is "any directly acting compound whose effects are stereospecifically antagonized by naloxone" [12]. In brief, opioids are all substances, whether natural or synthetic, which have morphinelike properties and bind specifically to opioid receptors.

In addition to analgesia, clinically useful opioids are capable of producing a wide variety of desired results as well as untoward effects pertaining to the respiratory system, gastrointestinal tract, cardiovascular system, mood, and rewarding processes. Depending on their opioid receptor effects, the opioids are divided into pure agonists, antagonists, and mixed agonists/antagonists, also called partial agonists [13]. When an agonist (eg, morphine) binds to the opioid receptor (eg, mu), it causes analgesia, euphoria, respiratory depression, and miosis. The potencies of various agonists differ

and therefore, so too do their doses for maximal therapeutic effect. For example, codeine is considered to be a weak agonist in that it needs to be given
at greater doses than morphine to achieve clinically comparable analgesic
effects. On the other hand, antagonists such as naloxone are capable of
blocking the effects of the agonists by occupying the receptor without acti-
vating it. Mixed or partial agonists are capable of stimulating the receptor.
However, because of their ability to compete with the full agonists for binding to the opioid receptor, they can actually reduce the final efficacy expected from an agonist. Therefore, the activity of a partial agonist
depends on the circumstance and could have mixed agonist and antagonist
activity. Interestingly, an opioid can act as agonist for one opioid receptor
type and antagonist for the other. Regardless, it is generally recognized
that the mu receptors, described in more detail later, are the mediators of
various desired and undesired effects generally expected of the opioid
therapeutics.

In general, the pharmacologic activity and therapeutic effects of various
opioids are compared with morphine. There are also several agonist and antagonist opioid drugs that are structurally related to morphine. A partial list
of these includes the agonists codeine, hydrocodone, hydromorphone, and
oxycodone; the antagonists naloxone and naltrexone; and the partial agonist
buprenorphine. Codeine is the most widely prescribed natural opioid (ie,
opiate) and its therapeutic effects are mediated by hepatic conversion to
morphine. A synthetic analog of codeine is tramadol, which in addition to
its weak opioid action, blocks the reuptake of other neurotransmitters
such as serotonin. Hydrocodone is synthesized from codeine and is considered to be more potent. On the other hand, hydromorphone, the active metabolite of hydrocodone, is 7 to 10 times more potent than morphine.
Interestingly, hydromorphone can be produced as a minor metabolite of
morphine in humans [14]. Both oxycodone and codeine are methylated at
position 3. Unlike morphine, there is better oral/parenteral relative analgesic
potency ratio for both of these opioids as compared with morphine [15].

Additional mu opioid receptor agonists available clinically include the
synthetic analogs including meperidine, fentanyl, methadone, and propoxyphene [11]. Meperidine and propoxyphene have less analgesic potency
compared with morphine, while methadone is comparable and fentanyl is
50 to 100 times more potent [16]. There are also several fentanyl analogs,
including sufentanil, which have several-fold greater potency than even
fentanyl [17]. In addition to the opioid receptor, the synthetic agonists
also bind to other types of receptors. Examples include methadone binding
to the N-methyl-D-aspartate (NMDA) receptor [18] and fentanyl releasing
noradrenaline, a phenomenon that is resistant to the naloxone antagonism
[19].

Morphine, tramadol, methadone, oxycodone, hydrocodone, and codeine
are all available as oral preparations. Morphine, hydromorphone, oxymor-
phone, and fentanyl can be administered intravenously. In addition,

fentanyl is frequently prescribed in the form of a patch at various strengths and oxycodone can be administered as a slow-release formulation [20]. As previously mentioned, some of these opioids are clinically available as combination products along with a nonopioid analgesic. Oxycodone combined with aspirin, ibuprofen, or acetaminophen is available in several different formulations and dosages, as are the combinations of codeine with acetaminophen or aspirin, hydrocodone with acetaminophen or ibuprofen, and tramadol with acetaminophen.

Hydrocodone is a semisynthetic opioid that is clinically used for both analgesic and antitussive properties. Hydrocodone elicits its pharmacologic activities through binding to the opioid receptors in the central nervous system. It appears that hydrocodone is a more effective opioid than codeine for relief of musculoskeletal pain [21] having six times the analgesic potency of codeine [22]. Hydrocodone is typically available as a combination product along with many other medications including nonopioid analgesics (eg, ibuprofen and acetaminophen), expectorants (eg, guaifenesin), decongestants (eg, pseudoephedrine), other cough suppressants (homatropine), and antihistamines (chlorpheniramine).

Many analgesic effectiveness studies involving combination drug formulations (an opioid combined with a nonopioid) have been reported. For example, in the treatment of moderate to severe postoperative obstetric or gynecologic pain, 2-tablet dose of hydrocodone 7.5 mg with ibuprofen 200 mg was comparable in efficacy to the 2-tablet dose of oxycodone 5 mg and acetaminophen 325 mg. Obviously both of these treatments were superior to the placebo [23]. In contrast, for treatment of chronic pain, the 2-tablet dose of hydrocodone 7.5 mg and ibuprofen 200 mg was more effective than either the 1-tablet dose of this combination or the 2-tablet dose of codeine 30 mg and acetaminophen 300 mg combination [24]. In a double-blind, randomized controlled trial involving 118 patients with chronic cancer pain, the combination formulation of hydrocodone (25 mg/d) and acetaminophen (2500 mg/d) was effective in relieving pain in 56.5% of the patients [25].

Clinical problems of opioid therapy

Adverse drug reactions

Pain management is plagued by two major factors: adverse drug reactions and undertreatment, as both patients and practitioners are fearful of addiction. Common side effects at conventional, therapeutic doses include somnolence, decreased gastric motility, nausea, vomiting, cutaneous flushing, and pruritis [11]. Although not typically life-threatening, these side effects represent quality of life issues for patients, often resulting in additional medications to alleviate the opioid side effects and increase compliance. At higher doses, opioids can cause miosis—pinpoint pupils that are pathognomonic of toxic doses—as well as mental changes, hearing loss [26], orthostatic hypotension, convulsions, and respiratory depression, the latter being the most common cause of opioid-related death [11]. Most of these adverse reactions, if recognized quickly, can be reversed upon administration of the opioid antagonist naloxone. Chronic opioid therapy can also lead to untoward hormonal effects. Suppression of sex hormones and cortisol can result in male and female infertility, decreased libido, and aggression, which can be reduced with specific hormone replacement therapies [27].

The availability of new routes of administration have led to increased utility and decreased opioid adverse drug reaction risk. Epidural and intrathecal administration through spinal catheters produces adequate regional analgesia at relatively low total doses compared with intravenous or oral routes. As such, spinal administration can thus minimize somnolence, nausea, vomiting, and respiratory depression associated with these medications. Other alternative routes include intranasal administration of butorphanol, and rectal and transdermal administration of fentanyl [28]. Availability of such options provides not only a decreased risk of adverse reactions, but also more comfortable measures for patients who would otherwise require continued intravenous administration, or for those who are unable to receive oral medication [28,29].

Undertreatment and fear of addiction

Physicians tend to prescribe pain medications conservatively, and patients and their families are often just as conservative, choosing to deal with some amount of pain rather than risk addiction. Indeed, the most common error made by physicians in managing severe pain is inadequate dosing of opioids [28]. As a result, many pain patients, including the terminally ill, suffer unnecessarily [28,30]. Lack of understanding of regulatory guidelines regarding the use of controlled substances and a social and legal environment that focuses on prescription drug abuse and a fear of unwanted regulatory scrutiny all contribute to the systemic practice of undertreating pain and the potential for erroneous identification of treatment-resistant patients as noncompliant or addicted [31].

Similar problems plague other therapies, such as warfarin anticoagulation, wherein concern about bleeding events leads to underdosing of that life-saving but potentially dangerous drug [32]. In the case of warfarin, undertreatment produces a high risk of blood clots and stroke [32], whereas the undertreatment of chronic pain decreases patients' functional status and quality of life, and can lead to loss of work, additional physical problems such as heart disease and obesity, an increased incidence of suicide, and an increased incidence of patients seeking illegal alternatives to alleviate their pain [31]. In both cases, pharmacogenetic diagnostics testing can be used to facilitate better understanding of the individual patient's risk, thereby freeing practitioners, armed with this knowledge, to practice medicine more effectively.

Fear of addiction leads to both undertreatment and noncompliance among opioid prescribers and patients, and part of this fear is a product of misunderstanding and misinterpretation of the symptoms of physical dependence and tolerance, one or both of which are characteristic effects of chronic opioid therapy (Fig. 1) [20,31]. Addiction is a primary chronic disease influenced by genetic, psychosocial, and environmental factors, and characterized by impaired control over drug use, compulsive use, continued use despite harm, and craving [1,20,31]. Two states of adaptation are physical dependence and tolerance. Physical dependence manifests as drug class–specific withdrawal symptoms as a result of abrupt cessation, rapid dose reduction, decreasing drug blood levels, and/or administration of an antagonist [1,31]. Tolerance is the condition in which exposure to a drug produces physiologic changes that cause the drug's effectiveness to be diminished over time [1,20,31]. Although the physical symptoms of withdrawal and the behavioral characteristics associated with physiologic tolerance (patients requesting increased drug dosages, complaints of persistent pain in spite of prescription compliance) are often interpreted as signs of addiction, it is important to note that tolerance and dependence are not equivalent with addiction, nor are they predictors of addiction development. The term "pseudoaddiction" has been defined to describe the iatrogenic result of physicians' misinterpretation of relief-seeking behaviors as the drug-seeking behaviors associated with addiction (see Fig. 1) [20,31]. Compounding the problem is the underappreciated and misunderstood contribution of genetics to the variability in patients' experience of pain (nociception), as well as their individual dose requirements and risk of experiencing the problems of

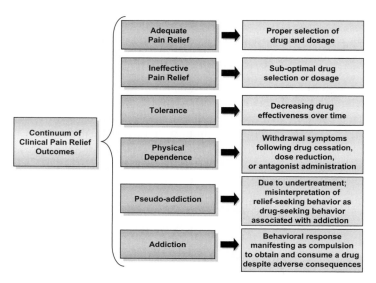

Fig. 1. Continuum of pain relief outcomes.

tolerance or addiction. Indeed, naïve patients whose genetics make them resistant to opioid therapy will experience little to no pain relief, and may quickly be judged noncompliant when in fact they are physiologically incapable of experiencing therapeutic benefit from the given drug.

A study from the American Pain Society estimates that 9% of the US adult population suffer from moderate to severe noncancer-related chronic pain [33]. More than half (57%) of these patients report severe to very severe pain, which is more likely to be constant than "flare-up," and less likely to be caused by arthritis [33]. In spite of reporting substantial pain, almost 40% are not currently seeing a physician for their pain, and those who are being treated by a physician are those who report experiencing severe (72%) and moderate (51%) pain [33]. Chronic pain sufferers who report moderate to severe pain are more likely to visit the emergency room, require hospitalization, or receive counseling for their pain [33]. As an indicator of the difficulty patients experience in obtaining effective pain relief, it is interesting to note that 47% of all chronic pain sufferers find it necessary to change doctors several times and their reasons for doing so include insufficient pain relief (42%), perceived lack of physician's knowledge or willingness to treat pain (27%–31%), and a perceived lack of sympathy (29%) [33]. Also telling is the fact that, although 55% of chronic pain sufferers report their pain as "under control," the vast majority of these (70%) are those reporting only moderate pain. The more severe a sufferer's pain, the less likely they are to consider their pain "under control" (51% severe, 39% very severe). When pain is under control, there are significant positive improvements in the sufferer's quality of life and emotional health, except in the case of very severe pain.

From a physician's standpoint, effective pain management is complicated by several factors, including (1) strict regulatory requirements and concerns about addiction or diversion, and (2) the fact that both the experience and treatment of pain are subject to a broad degree of interindividual variability. The House of Delegates of the Federation of State Medical Boards of the United States cites several major contributors to the problem of pain undertreatment [31]. Topping the list is a lack of knowledge among practitioners regarding medical standards, the latest research, and clinical guidelines for administering appropriate pain treatment; this lack of knowledge contributes to a misunderstanding of the disparate concepts of dependence and addiction. Many practitioners, unfamiliar with regulatory processes and policies, are also unsettled by the perception that prescribing adequate amounts of controlled substances to effect pain relief will trigger regulatory scrutiny [31]. Although pain policies and procedures are being put in place by state medical boards, the implementation and adoption of such policies is not uniform and can vary substantially between jurisdictions. Setting such policy and procedural issues aside, the very subjective nature of pain is at the heart of the problem for practitioners. Research has found that the experience of pain and patients' response to therapy (with regard to adverse reactions and therapeutic benefit), are subject to wide interindividual variability caused by a number of factors, including patient age, organ function, comedication, underlying disease, and genetics.

Current chronic pain management guidelines suggest a multidisciplinary, or biopsychosocial, model that incorporates pharmacologic and psychologic approaches to treating pain. Even acute pain management guidelines, such as those for postsurgical patients, incorporate various psychosocial elements in addition to general pharmacologic approaches. Although guidelines may call for titration protocols and pharmacovigilance for such adverse reactions as excessive sedation and respiratory depression, they are all based on a general "try it and see" approach; patient therapy is generally initiated using a standard drug and dosage that is typically based on a patient's reported pain level as measured on a standardized pain scale. Although these methods are meant to assist physicians in tailoring pain management to the needs of the individual patient, these are all based on inherently subjective measures. Not only do these subjective approaches create a lack of clarity for physicians as they approach patient management, they also can lead to misunderstandings when standard therapeutic protocols appear to fail. Adverse reactions are events to which physicians currently must respond after the fact, as they have no tools available to them to avoid or alleviate the risk. Patients who report no pain relief can also present a confounding element to physicians, in the absence of any evidence as to the cause for the therapeutic failure. In many such cases, the patient's particular genetic profile may present some explanation.

Pharmacogenetic effects on opioid sensitivity

The genetic effects on patient drug sensitivity (ie, therapeutic response and relative risk of experiencing adverse effects) can be separated into two mechanistic categories: pharmacokinetics and pharmacodynamics. A patient's metabolic status, or their ability to metabolize certain drugs, affects the drug pharmacokinetics. For example, a patient with impaired metabolism may be unable to activate a prodrug such as codeine into the active morphine metabolite. Such patients will report little to no pain relief in response to codeine therapy, and may not receive therapeutic benefit even from greater dosages. In other cases, a patient may metabolize the prodrug excessively quickly, and is thus at greater risk for toxicity. A patient's ability to respond to a drug is also determined at the level of the drug target, or receptor, also referred to as pharmacodynamics. Patients exhibit genetic variability in the number and functional status of their receptors, which leads to interindividual variability in therapeutic response to certain drug therapies. For example, a patient who has a nonfunctional receptor for a certain drug will be unable to respond to that drug regardless of the dosage. Patients with varying degrees of receptor functionality may require different dosages than patients exhibiting no such variable.

In the case of opioid analgesic therapies, several pharmacokinetic and pharmacodynamic players have been identified as reliable indicators of therapeutic efficacy with regard to certain drugs. The cytochrome P450 metabolic enzymes have been implicated in the metabolism of opioid drugs, and variants in these enzymes, specifically the CYP2D6 and CYP2C19, have been linked to toxicity and therapeutic efficacy of opioids. In addition, opioid receptors, specifically the mu and kappa opioid receptors, have been implicated both in the therapeutic efficacy and the risk of experiencing adverse effects. Of these biomarkers, CYP2D6 and OPRM1 (the mu1 opioid receptor) have been thus far identified as having the greatest relevance to determining a patient's relative risk of experiencing adverse effects and the potential therapeutic efficacy of opioid therapies (Table 1). These are discussed further in the following sections.

Opioid Metabolism by CYP2D6

CYP2D6 catalyzes the biotransformation of several opioid prodrugs into their active metabolies. These include codeine, dihydrocodeine, oxycodone, hydrocodone, tramadol, dextropropoxyphene, ethylmorphine, and to some extent, methadone. For example, approximately 90% of a codeine dose is metabolized to inactive metabolites by CYP3A4, which undergo subsequent conjugation and renal elimination. The other 10% of a codeine dose undergoes O-demethylation by CYP2D6 and accounts for the analgesic activity of the medication (Fig. 2) [34]. Glucuronidation of morphine to morphine-6-glucuronide produces an additional active metabolite. Hydrocodone is also metabolized to the more potent hydromorphone by CYP2D6 O-demethylation, in addition to other pathways including N-demethylation to norhydrocodone and 6-keto reduction to the corresponding hydroxy-metabolites (hydrocodol) and hydromorphol [22].

Phenotypic differences in CYP2D6 metabolizer status, as a function of genotype, are categorized as poor, intermediate, extensive, and ultra-rapid. These phenotypic categories and the most common pharmacogenetic polymorphisms associated with the designations are more broadly described in other articles in this issue (see the articles by de Leon and colleagues and Algeciras-Schimnich and colleagues) [35–37]. Briefly, CYP2D6 poor metabolizers (PM) are those who have two deficient alleles, found in approximately 7% to 10% of white populations and 1% to 2% in African Americans. They are unable to metabolize most opioids, antidepressants, and antipsychotics, and are therefore prone to experiencing elevated blood concentrations of those medications. In addition, because of the lack of CYP2D6 activity, PMs are also unable to convert certain prodrugs into their active metabolites, eg, codeine to morphine or tamoxifen to endoxifen, resulting in therapeutic failure from administration of the inactive parent compound [37,38]. For example, PMs administered hydrocodone will produce little to no active hydromorphone and are at risk of analgesic failure

Table 1
Clinical effects of CYP2D6 and OPRM1 variants on opioid toxicity and efficacy

Gene	Gene variants	Opioid	Effect	Clinical consequence
Pharmacokinetic variants				
CYP2D6	Inactive alleles: *3–*7, and others Partially active alleles: *9, *10, *17, *41	Codeine	Decreased morphine production via O-demethylation	Loss of opioid analgesia
		Tramadol	Decreased O-desmethyl tramadol production	Slightly decreased analgesia and increased side effects
		Oxycodone	Decreased oxymorphone production	Decreased analgesia and increased side effects
		Hydrocodone	Decreased hydromorphone production	Unclear; no significant effects
	Ultra-rapid alleles: *1xN, *2xN (active allele duplication)	Codeine	Increased morphine production	Increased morphine effects and risk of ADRs
		Oxycodone	Increased oxymorphone production	Increased risk of ADRs
		Hydrocodone	Increased hydromorphone production	Increased risk of ADRs
Pharmacodynamic variants				
OPRM1	118A > G	Morphine and Alfentanil	Unclear; impaired receptor affinity, and possibly decreased expression	Decreased effectiveness, increased dose requirement

Abbreviations: CYP2D6, cytochrome P450 2D6; OPRM1, mu opioid receptor 1; ADR, adverse drug reaction.
Data from Refs [53,60–62].

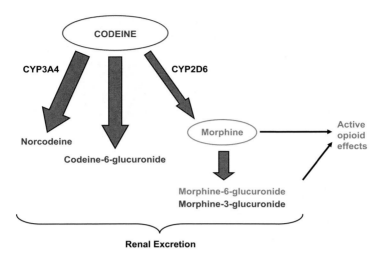

Fig. 2. Codeine metabolism. Roughly 90% of a codeine dose is metabolized to inactive compounds by CYP3A4. The other 10% of a codeine dose is metabolized to the active component morphine via CYP2D6. All are eventually excreted by the kidneys. Blue, inactive compounds; red, active metabolites.

[35,39]. Previous pharmacokinetic studies have shown after taking a single oral does of 10 mg hydrocodone, extensive metabolizers (EMs) display peak serum hydromorphone concentrations roughly five times that of the PMs [39]. Further, the mean peak serum concentrations in PMs are consistent with serum hydromorphone concentrations in patients who received the same 10-mg hydrocodone dose together with the strong CYP2D6 inhibitor quinidine, thus demonstrating how CYP2D6 metabolic capacity is the determinant for therapeutic hydromorphone concentrations. By leveraging these single-dose peak serum hydromorphone concentration data, the effect of PM status on chronic hydrocodone dosing can be modeled (Fig. 3). Using standard pharmacokinetic calculations for the concentration maximum at steady state ($Cmax_{ss}$) following 10-mg hydrocodone dosing every 6 hours, it is clear that PMs consistently produce no appreciable hydromorphone concentrations as compared with EMs (see Fig. 3). Whether the difference in serum drug concentrations results in differential analgesic efficacy remains to be determined.

Intermediate metabolizers (IMs) are typically defined as those who carry one deficient allele and one active allele, or two partially deficient alleles [36,40,41]. These individuals retain some residual capacity to metabolize drugs, but are still at risk of experiencing somewhat elevated blood levels and associated side effects at standard dosages [36,40,41]. EMs are considered "normal," and are homozygous for the wild-type or common allele. These individuals retain full metabolic capacity, and in general, receive benefit from standard dosages of medications that are CYP2D6 substrates.

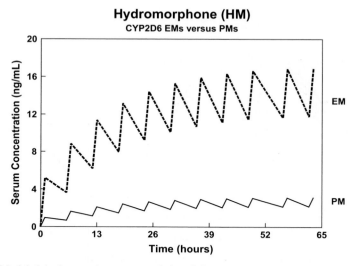

Fig. 3. Modeled hydromorphone accumulation following repeated hydrocodone dosing as a function of CYP2D6 metabolizer status. Hydromorphone concentrations calculated are approximately five times higher in EMs compared with PMs following 10-mg hydrocodone dosing every 6 hours, based on genotype-specific peak hydromorphone serum concentrations [39]. EM, extensive metabolizer; PM, poor metabolizer.

In contrast, ultra-rapid metabolizers (UMs) carry three or more functional alleles, and are present in 1% to 2% of whites and up to 29% of Northern African populations. These patients metabolize drugs much more quickly, and may see little or no therapeutic benefit from standard dosages, as they eliminate the drug too quickly to allow therapeutic drug concentrations to be achieved. Or, in the case of a prodrug such as codeine, UMs may achieve higher than normal blood concentrations of the active metabolite morphine, thus putting these patients at risk of toxic side effects [33,42]. A recent case report detailed the fatal morphine overdose of a breast-feeding neonate whose mother, a CYP2D6 UM, had been taking low-dose codeine for episiotomy pain. Postmortem analysis of the baby's blood and mother's stored breast milk showed morphine levels well over 10 times higher than would have been expected in both fluids [43]. This case report led to the Food and Drug Administration (FDA) public health advisory issued in August 2007 informing health care professionals about the safety of codeine-based products given to breastfeeding mothers who are CYP2D6 UMs [44]. In the advisory, the FDA warned that higher levels of morphine in the breast milk of UM mothers prescribed codeine can lead to life-threatening or fatal side effects in nursing babies, and that doctors should educate their nursing patients how to recognize signs of morphine overdose. The FDA subsequently asked makers of codeine-based pharmaceuticals to include information about metabolic differences and breastfeeding concerns in the drug labels. Although this situation has been reported only with co-deine, the FDA notes that it has the potential to affect other narcotics with active metabolites produced by CYP2D6, and, thus, cause the same se-rious side effects in nursing infants if the breast milk drug levels are high [44].

Opioid response via μ-opioid receptor

Opioid receptors

Opioid receptors are members of the G-protein–coupled transmembrane protein class [45]. They are present throughout both central and peripheral nervous systems and are linked to various neurotransmitter systems. In the mid-1970s, Martin and colleagues [46] proposed the idea of multiple opioid receptor subtypes with ligands having agonist, antagonist, or mixed agonist activity. The list of opioid receptor subtypes has been growing in part be-cause of the identification of their endogenous ligands such as enkephalins, endorphins, and dynorphin [45] as well as the availability of selective ago-nists and antagonists.

There are nomenclature schemes for various subtypes of opioid receptors. One very traditional and popular approach has been the use of Greek letters to refer to the drug that was used in the study of that particular receptor subtype [12]. For example, mu (μ) stands for morphine, kappa (κ) for ketocyclazocine, sigma (σ) for SKF-10,047, also known as N-allylnor-metazocine, and delta (δ) for deferens. The sigma was later shown to be nonopioid in nature; therefore, the mu, kappa, and delta are the pharmaco-logically defined opioid receptors [12,47]. Additional receptors including ep-silon (ε), zeta (ζ), and lambda (λ) have also been described [12]. An alternative approach to naming opioid receptors is the use of the OP series starting from that which was described first (ie, delta), OP_1. This was fol-lowed by OP_2 and OP_3 for kappa and mu receptors, respectively. Molecular biologists have also used their own nomenclature referring to delta, kappa, and mu as *DOR, KOR,* and *MOR* receptors, respectively. For most clini-cians, the original Greek alphabet system is the most familiar.

Regardless of the nomenclature used, it is evident that opioid receptors have structural similarity, but each has distinct clinical effects and tissue dis-tribution. In addition to the classical opioid receptors, a new G-protein–coupled receptor signaling system referred to as the opioid-receptor-like 1 (ORL1) receptor has been cloned [48]. Significant structural-functional ho-mology as well as positive cooperativity between the two systems has been described [48]. Nociceptin, an endogenous ligand for ORL1, is a nonopioid peptide able to modulate pain response [49]. However, it is evident that most of the currently available opioid therapeutic analgesics exert their analgesic and adverse effects primarily through the classical mu receptors [50]. The ag-onists of the mu opioid receptor share many pharmacologic characteristics that now are known to be mediated through the subtypes of this receptor.

Cloning experiments of MOR-1 have suggested that there are at least seven splice variants of this gene leading to the variability in analgesic effects of opioids with mu receptor affinity [51]. Interestingly, each of these variants selectively binds morphine and other drugs that act at the MOR receptor (currently referred to as mu opioid peptide or MOP). For example, naloxonazine antagonizes the mu-1 whereas morphine-6-beta-gluruconide affects the mu-2 subtype. The other opioid receptors including delta and kappa also have various subtypes, which will not be discussed here.

μ-opioid receptor genotyping

Opioid agonists, such as morphine, hydromorphone, and fentanyl, exert their analgesic properties via stimulation of the mu receptors. Their analgesic effects increase in a log-linear fashion with the dose, although this theoretically unlimited effect is tempered by the occurrence of increasingly intolerable side effects, which are also mediated by the mu receptors. Analgesic efficacy of mu-acting drugs has been linked to the 118A > G single nucleotide polymorphism (SNP) of OPRM1, the gene encoding the mu-1 receptor. The frequency of the variant G allele varies from 10% to 48% depending on the population studied [52]. The base substitution creates a missense mutation in the N-terminus of the protein, changing an asparagine to aspartic acid. This results in the loss of a site (one of five) for receptor N-glycosylation. The polymorphism in OPRM1 has also been reported to affect the expression of the mu receptor [53]. Early reports that the variant affects receptor binding potential have not been confirmed, leaving the precise mechanism for the variant's effect a mystery [54,55]. The polymorphism has been found to affect both nociception and the therapeutic efficacy of opioid drugs [56,57].

Studies show that patients carrying the GG (homozygous variant) genotype require much higher opioid doses to achieve pain relief [58,59]. In one study, OPRM1 AA patients required an average dose of 112 mg morphine/24 hrs, AG patients required 132 mg morphine/24 hrs, and GG patients required 216 mg morphine/24 hrs [58]. The difference between these groups' pain scores was not statistically significant during therapy, indicating that pain relief was consistent across the variable dose ranges and genotype groups. Another study of cancer patients found a similar difference between the morphine dose requirements of AA (97 mg/24 hrs) and GG (225 mg/24 hrs) patients, but did not see the same intermediate dose requirement for the heterozygous group (66 mg/24 hrs) [59]. In this study, however, the median pain score for this group was significantly different from the others.

When one considers such drastically different dose requirements for patients carrying the GG genotype and the frequency of the genotype, it is not surprising that many patients receiving standard dosing regimens frequently complain of insufficient opioid pain relief. Thus, the use of the OPRM1 118A > G variant as a diagnostic marker could facilitate the identification of patients who may be less sensitive (or, more resistant) to standard opioid therapeutic regimens, and may help guide individualized dosing and therapeutic choices.

Summary

Adequate pain management in the United States represents a significant ongoing problem facing physicians, patients, and regulatory agencies. The use of opioids continues to be a mainstay of pain management strategies, despite their risks of toxicity and addiction; thus, more effective means by which to provide adequate pain relief while balancing the potential negative aspects is paramount. Integration of novel diagnostics, such as the pharmacogenetic biomarkers CYP2D6 and OPRM1, hold promise as a means by which to assess a patient's risk of adverse events or likelihood of efficacy. With a priori knowledge of a patient's potential for beneficial response to a given opioid, a physician is armed with critical information that can guide therapeutic decisions in real time. Incorporation of such biomarkers are emerging on the forefront of personalized medicine, and have the potential to dramatically improve the utility and efficacy of both current and future pain management strategies.

References

[1] Rasor J, Harris G. Using opioids for patients with moderate to severe pain. J Am Osteopath Assoc 2007;107(9 Suppl 5):ES4–10.
[2] Pain in the workplace—a 10-year update of Ortho-McNeil's survey on the impact of pain on the workplace. Titusville (NJ): PriCara, Unit of Ortho-McNeil Pharmaceutical Inc.; 2006.
[3] Stewart WF, Ricci JA, Chee E, et al. Lost productive time and cost due to common pain conditions in the US workforce. JAMA 2003;290:2443–54.
[4] Ventafridda V, Saita L, Ripamonti C, et al. WHO guidelines for the use of analgesics in cancer pain. Int J Tissue React 1985;7:93–6.
[5] Sepulveda C, Marlin A, Yoshida T, et al. Palliative care: the World Health Organization's global perspective. J Pain Symptom Manage 2002;24:91–6.
[6] Jadad AR, Browman GP. The WHO analgesic ladder for cancer pain management. Stepping up the quality of its evaluation. JAMA 1995;274:1870–3.
[7] Azevedo SL, Ferreira K, Kimura M, et al. The WHO analgesic ladder for cancer pain control, twenty years of use. How much pain relief does one get from using it? Support Care Cancer 2006;14:1086–93.
[8] Krenzischek DA, Dunwoody CJ, Polomano RC, et al. Pharmacotherapy for acute pain: implications for practice. J Perianesth Nurs 2008;23:S28–42.
[9] Gajraj NM. COX-2 inhibitors celecoxib and parecoxib: valuable options for postoperative pain management. Curr Top Med Chem 2007;7:235–49.
[10] Martinez-Gonzalez J, Badimon L. Mechanisms underlying the cardiovascular effects of COX-inhibition: benefits and risks. Curr Pharm Des 2007;13:2215–27.
[11] Gutstein HB, Akil H. Opioid analgesics. In: Brunton LL, Lazo JS, Parker KL, editors. Goodman and Gilman's the pharmacological basis of therapeutics. 11th edition. New York: McGraw-Hill; 2006. p. 547–90.
[12] Dhawan BN, Cesselin F, Raghubir R, et al. International union of pharmacology. XII. Classification of opioid receptors. Pharmacol Rev 1996;48:567–92.

[13] Schlaepfer TE, Strain EC, Greenberg BD, et al. Site of opioid action in the human brain: mu and kappa agonists' subjective and cerebral blood flow effects. Am J Psychiatry 1998;155:470–3.

[14] Cone EJ, Heit HA, Caplan YH, et al. Evidence of morphine metabolism to hydromorphone in pain patients chronically treated with morphine. J Anal Toxicol 2006;30:1–5.

[15] Beaver WT, Wallenstein SL, Rogers A, et al. Analgesic studies of codeine and oxycodone in patients with cancer. I. Comparisons of oral with intramuscular codeine and of oral with intramuscular oxycodone. J Pharmacol Exp Ther 1978;207:92–100.

[16] Clotz MA, Nahata MC. Clinical uses of fentanyl, sufentanil, and alfentanil. Clin Pharm 1991;10:581–93.

[17] Willens JS, Myslinski NR. Pharmacodynamics, pharmacokinetics, and clinical uses of fentanyl, sufentanil, and alfentanil. Heart Lung 1993;22:239–51.

[18] Gorman AL, Elliott KJ, Inturrisi CE. The d- and l-isomers of methadone bind to the noncompetitive site on the N-methyl-D-aspartate (NMDA) receptor in rat forebrain and spinal cord. Neurosci Lett 1997;223:5–8.

[19] Atcheson R, Rowbotham DJ, Lambert DG. Fentanyl inhibits the release of [3H]noradrenaline from SH-SY5Y human neuroblastoma cells. Br J Anaesth 1994;72:98–103.

[20] Galvagno AM, Correll DJ, Narang S. Safe oral equianalgesic opioid dosing for patients with moderate to severe pain. Resid Staff Physician 2007;53(4):17–25.

[21] Turturro MA, Paris PM, Yealy DM, et al. Hydrocodone versus codeine in acute musculoskeletal pain. Ann Emerg Med 1991;20:1100–3.

[22] Baselt RC, editor. Disposition of toxic drugs and chemicals in man. 7th edition. Foster City: Biomedical Publications; 2004. p. 546.

[23] Palangio M, Wideman GL, Keffer M, et al. Combination hydrocodone and ibuprofen versus combination oxycodone and acetaminophen in the treatment of postoperative obstetric or gynecologic pain. Clin Ther 2000;22:600–12.

[24] Palangio M, Damask MJ, Morris E, et al. Combination hydrocodone and ibuprofen versus combination codeine and acetaminophen for the treatment of chronic pain. Clin Ther 2000; 22:879–92.

[25] Rodriguez RF, Castillo JM, Castillo MP, et al. Hydrocodone/acetaminophen and tramadol chlorhydrate combination tablets for the management of chronic cancer pain: a double-blind comparative trial. Clin J Pain 2008;24:1–4.

[26] Friedman RA, House JW, Luxford WM, et al. Profound hearing loss associated with hydrocodone/acetaminophen abuse. Am J Otol 2000;21:188–9.

[27] Ballantyne JC. Opioid analgesia: perspectives on right use and utility. Pain Physician 2007; 10:479–91.

[28] Fields HL, Martin JB. Pain: pathophysiology and management. In: Fauci AS, Braunwald E, Kasper DL, editors. Harrison's principles of internal medicine. 17th edition. New York: McGraw-Hill; 2008. p. 81–7.

[29] Vallerand AH. The use of long-acting opioids in chronic pain management. Nurs Clin North Am 2003;38(3):435–45.

[30] SUPPORT study principal investigators. A controlled trial to improve care for seriously ill hospitalized patients. JAMA 1995;274(20):1591–8.

[31] Gilson AM, Joranson DE, Mauer MA. Improving medical board policies: influence of a model. J Law Med Ethics 2003;31:128.

[32] Reynolds KK, Valdes R Jr, Hartung BR, et al. Individualizing warfarin therapy. Pers Med 2007;4(1):11–31.

[33] Starch R. Chronic pain in America: roadblocks to relief. Amer Acad Pain Med, Amer Pain Soc, and Janssen Pharmaceutica 1999.

[34] Gasche Y, Daali Y, Fathi M, et al. Codeine intoxication associated with ultrarapid CYP2D6 metabolism. N Engl J Med 2004;351(27):2827–31.

[35] Lurcott G. The effects of the genetic absence and inhibition of CYP2D6 on the metabolism of codeine and its derivatives hydrocodone and oxycodone. Anesth Prog 1999;45:154–6.

[36] Linder MW, Evans WE, McLeod HL. Application of pharmacogenetic principles to clinical pharmacology. In: Burton ME, editor. Applied pharmacokinetics & pharmacodynamics: principles of therapeutic drug monitoring. Baltimore (MD): Lippincott Williams & Wilkins; 2005. p. 165–85.

[37] Foster A, Mobley E, Wang X. Complicated pain management in a CYP2D6 poor metabolizer. Pain Pract 2007;7(4):352–6.

[38] Caraco Y, Sheller J, Wood AJJ. Pharmacogenetic determination of the effects of codeine and prediction of drug interactions. J Pharmacol Exp Ther 1996;278(3):1165–74.

[39] Otton AV, Schadel M, Cheung SW, et al. CYP2D6 phenotype determines the metabolic conversion of hydrocodone to hydromorphone. Clin Pharmacol Ther 1993;54(5):463–72.

[40] Kirchheiner J, Brøsen K, Dahl ML, et al. CYP2D6 and CYP2C19 genotype-based dose recommendations for antidepressants: a first step towards subpopulation-specific dosages. Acta Psychiatr Scand 2001;104(3):173–92.

[41] Kirchheiner J, Nickchen K, Bauer M, et al. Pharmacogenetics of antidepressants and antipsychotics: the contribution of allelic variations to the phenotype of drug response. Mol Psychiatry 2004;9(5):442–73.

[42] Kirchheiner J, Schmidt H, Tzvetkov M, et al. Pharmacokinetics of codeine and its metabolite morphine in ultra-rapid metabolizers due to CYP2D6 duplication. Pharmacogenomics 2007; 7:257–65.

[43] Koren G, Cairns J, Chitayat D, et al. Pharmacogenetics of morphine poisoning in a breastfed neonate of a codeine-prescribed mother. Lancet 2006;368(9536):704.

[44] U.S. Food and Drug Administration. Use of codeine by some breastfeeding mothers may lead to life-threatening side effects in nursing babies. FDA Public Health Advisory 2007, Avaliable at: http://www.fda.gov/CDER/Drug/advisory/codeine.htm. Accessed October 10, 2008.

[45] Piestrzeniewicz MK, Fichna J, Janecka A. Opioid receptors and their selective ligands. Postepy Biochem 2006;52:313–9.

[46] Martin WR, Eades CG, Thompson JA, et al. The effects of morphine- and nalorphine-like drugs in the nondependent and morphine-dependent chronic spinal dog. J Pharmacol Exp Ther 1976;197:517–32.

[47] Steinfels GF, Alberici GP, Tam SW, et al. Biochemical, behavioral, and electrophysiologic actions of the selective sigma receptor ligand (+)-pentazocine. Neuropsychopharmacology 1998;1:321–7.

[48] New DC, Wong YH. The ORL1 receptor: molecular pharmacology and signalling mechanisms. Neurosignals 2002;11:197–212.

[49] Yeon KY, Sim MY, Choi SY, et al. Molecular mechanisms underlying calcium current modulation by nociceptin. Neuroreport 2004;15:2205–9.

[50] Ananthan S. Opioid ligands with mixed mu/delta opioid receptor interactions: an emerging approach to novel analgesics. AAPS J 2006;8:E118–25.

[51] Pasternak GW. Insights into mu opioid pharmacology: the role of mu opioid receptor subtypes. Life Sci 2001;68:2213–9.

[52] Kreek MJ, Bart G, Lilly C, et al. Pharmacogenetics and human molecular genetics of opiate and cocaine addictions and their treatments. Pharmacol Rev 2005;57(1):1–26.

[53] Zhang Y, Wang D, Johnson AD, et al. Allelic expression imbalance of human mu opioid receptor (OPRM1) caused by variant A118G. J Biolumin Chemilumin 2005;280: 32618–24.

[54] Bond C, LaForge KS, Tian M, et al. Single-nucleotide polymorphism in the human mu opioid receptor gene alters beta-endorphin binding and activity: possible implications for opiate addiction. Proc Natl Acad Sci U S A 1998;95(16):9608–13.

[55] Beyer A, Koch T, Schroder H, et al. Effect of the A118G polymorphism on binding affinity, potency and agonist-mediated endocytosis, desensitization, and resensitization of the human mu-opioid receptor. J Neurochem 2004;89:553–60.

[56] Fillingim RB, Kaplan L, Staud R, et al. The A118G single nucleotide polymorphism of the mu-opioid receptor gene (OPRM1) is associated with pressure pain sensitivity in humans. J Pain 2005;6:159–67.

[57] Lotsch J, Geisslinger G. Relevance of frequent mu-opioid receptor polymorphisms for opioid activity in healthy volunteers. Pharmacogenomics 2006;6(3):200–10.

[58] Reyes-Gibby CC, Shete S, Rakvåg T, et al. Exploring joint effects of genes and the clinical efficacy of morphine for cancer pain: OPRM1 and COMT gene. Pain 2007;130(1–2):25–30.

[59] Klepstad P, Rakvåg TT, Kaasa S, et al. The 118A > G polymorphism in the human mu-opioid receptor gene may increase morphine requirements in patients with pain caused by malignant disease. Acta Anaesthesiol Scand 2004;48(10):1232–9.

[60] Lotsch J, Skarke C, Liefhold J, et al. Genetic predictors of the clinical response to opioid analgesics. Clin Pharm 2004;43(14):983–1013.

[61] de Leon J, Dinsmore L, Wedlund P. Adverse drug reactions to oxycodone and hydrocodone in CYP2D6 ultrarapid metabolizers. J Clin Psychopharmacol 2003;23(4):420–1.

[62] Susce MT, Murray-Carmichael E, de Leon J. Response to hydrocodone, codeine, and oxycodone in a CYP2D6 poor metabolizer. Prog Neuropsychopharmacol Biol Psychiatry 2006; 30(7):1356–8.

ELSEVIER
SAUNDERS

CLINICS IN
LABORATORY
MEDICINE

Clin Lab Med 28 (2008) 599–617

Pharmacogenetic Testing in Psychiatry: A Review of Features and Clinical Realities

José de Leon, MD[a,b,c,*], Maria J. Arranz, PhD[d],
Gualberto Ruaño, MD, PhD[e]

[a]*University of Kentucky Mental Health Research Center at Eastern State Hospital,*
627 West Fourth Street, Lexington, KY 40508, USA
[b]*University of Kentucky Colleges of Medicine and Pharmacy, Lexington, KY 40536, USA*
[c]*Institute of Neurosciences, University of Granada, Granada, E-18071 Spain*
[d]*Senior Lecturer, Clinical Neuropsychopharmacology, Psychological Medicine, Institute of Psychiatry,*
King's College, PO 51, Room N2.07, 1, Windsor Walk, London SE5 8AF, UK
[e]*CEO, Genomas, Inc., 67 Jefferson Street, Hartford, CT 06106, USA*

Five pharmacogenetic tests are described in detail in this article. To avoid biases due to conflict of interest, only peer-reviewed articles were used for the data discussed. The AmpliChip CYP450 Test is marketed by Roche Molecular Systems, Inc. Dr. de Leon received researcher-initiated grants ending in 2007 from Roche Molecular Systems, Inc. He was on Roche Molecular Systems, Inc.'s Advisory Board in 2006. His lectures have been supported seven times by Roche Molecular Systems, Inc. (one in 2005 and six in 2006). He has never been a consultant to, and has no other financial arrangements with, Roche Molecular Systems, Inc. Other coauthors have no conflict of interest with Roche Molecular Systems, Inc. The Tag-It Mutation Detection Kit is marketed by Luminex. Dr. Ruaño's laboratory uses this test. Other coauthors have no conflict of interest with Luminex. The LGC clozapine response test was developed in part by Dr. Arranz. She actively collaborates with LGC in the development of genetic tests and has received consultant fees from LGC. Other coauthors have no conflict of interest with LGC. The PGxPredict:Clozapine was marketed by PGxHealth. The authors have no conflict of interest with PGxHealth. The PhyzioType system is proprietary to Genomas. Dr. Ruaño is the CEO of Genomas and is supported by the NIH Small Business Innovation Research Grant 2 R44 MH073291-02 "DNA Diagnostics for Minimizing Metabolic Side-Effects of Antipsychotics." Dr. de Leon is a coinvestigator for this NIH grant. He has never been a consultant to, and has no other financial arrangements with, Genomas. Dr. Arranz has no relationship with Genomas, but was a coauthor of one of the articles using The PhyzioType system in which Dr. de Leon was the first author.

Dr. de Leon has received researcher-initiated grants from Eli Lilly as a co-investigator (completed in 2007) and as the investigator (completed in 2000). He was on the advisory boards of Bristol-Myers Squibb (2003/04) and AstraZeneca (2003). He personally develops his presentations for lecturing and has never lectured using any pharmaceutic company presentations. His lectures have been supported three times by Eli Lilly (one in 2003 and two in 2006), twice by Janssen (2000 and 2006), twice by Pfizer (both in 2001), once by Bristol-Myers Squibb (2006), twice by Lundbeck (both in 1999), and once by Sandoz (1997). He has never been a consultant to, and has no other financial arrangements with, pharmacogenetic or pharmaceutical companies nor owns any of their stocks. Dr. Arranz, PhD, is a consultant for TheraGenetics (UK), a company she cofounded and that is dedicated to the development of pharmacogenetic tests.

* Corresponding author. Mental Health Research Center at Eastern State Hospital, 627 West Fourth Street, Lexington, KY 40508.
E-mail address: jdeleon@uky.edu (J. de Leon).

0272-2712/08/$ - see front matter © 2008 Elsevier Inc. All rights reserved.
doi:10.1016/j.cll.2008.05.003 *labmed.theclinics.com*

Pharmacogenetics and personalized medicine

The development of new technologies at the end of the twentieth century [1] that permit parallel genetic testing (testing for many genetic variations), and the mapping of the human genome in 2000 [2], have brought hope that a new era in medicine is dawning [3]. The importance of these new technologies can be recognized when we remember that the human genome may have more than 20,000 genes and millions of variations, including the so-called single nucleotide polymorphism (SNP). More recently, some investigators have stressed that other types of genetic variations, such as deletions or duplications, the so-called copy number variations (CNV), may have been neglected [4].

A major technological breakthrough was the introduction of the Affymetrix GeneChip [1], a DNA microarray that allowed parallel genetic testing by introducing microchip technology. This technology has expanded to testing RNA and protein arrays and arrays including DNA, RNA, and proteins that are used in medical research. Currently, more advanced forms of these types of DNA microarray technologies allow the testing of more than a half million SNPs for less than $1000 per patient sample, and the cost is still declining.

The development of genomic medicine and genetic testing has helped in diagnosing some rare and unusual disorders. Potentially much more important is the field of pharmacogenetics or pharmacogenomics, which has been proposed as the driving force for implementing genetic medicine in primary care [5,6]. Roses [7] made an important distinction between two types of pharmacogenetics, that of safety pharmacogenetics to prevent adverse drug reactions and efficacy pharmacogenetics to predict response. A term related to pharmacogenetics used by lay journals is "personalized prescription," defined by *Science* [8] as "tailoring drugs to a patient's genetic makeup." This *Science* editorial in 1997 [8] predicted that personalized prescription will "soon" reach clinical practice. More precise estimations for the generalized use of personalized prescriptions have been provided: 2015 according to *Time* [9] magazine and 2020 according to *JAMA: The Journal of the American Medical Association* [10]. If the estimations for generalized medical use of personalized medicine are going to occur in 8 to 13 years, one should take note of the preliminary steps already occurring. Even business journals [11] reflect psychiatry's place at the forefront of the use of pharmacogenetics in medicine.

This article focuses on the first generation of pharmacogenetic tests that are potentially useful in psychiatry. Five pharmacogenetic tests are reviewed in detail. After reviewing these five tests, three practical aspects of implementing pharmacogenetic testing in psychiatric clinical practice are reviewed: (1) the evaluation of these tests in clinical practice, (2) cost-effectiveness, and (3) regulatory oversight. Finally, the future of these and other pharmacogenetic tests in psychiatry is discussed.

Pharmacogenetic tests in psychiatry

This article focuses on published information on the pharmacogenetic tests currently on the market or soon to be marketed. PubMed does not have a computer search strategy that provides information on marketed pharmacogenetic tests in psychiatry. Therefore, the authors, who have paid close attention to this area for the last 10 years and have extensively reviewed the literature [12–21], have made an effort, based on their experience, to describe all pharmacogenetic tests in psychiatry that have some information published in peer-reviewed journal articles or abstracts. The authors know that Pathway Diagnostics [22] and the Mayo Clinic Laboratory [23] offer tests to genotype for serotonin receptors and transporters. They have no published articles on their tests that are based on prior published literature that has been reviewed by Kirchheiner and colleagues [24]. If other unidentified pharmacogenetic tests in psychiatry have no published information, they may have been overlooked.

Four types of published pharmacogenetic tests are currently on the market, were previously on the market, or are ready to be introduced in the marketplace, which are potentially useful in psychiatry. First, a group of pharmacogenetic tests targets the cytochrome P450 (CYP); two of them receive additional attention in this article. They are the AmpliChip CYP450 Test [25,26] (developed by Roche Molecular Systems, Inc. [27], the first pharmacogenetic test [28] approved by the US Food and Drug Administration [FDA]) and the Luminex Tag-It Mutation Detection Kit [29–31] (developed originally by TM Bioscience, which was acquired by Luminex) [32], which has not yet been presented for FDA approval.

The second type is a pharmacogenetic test focused on clozapine efficacy [33]; it combines genetic variants of the neurotransmitter genes (clozapine response test) [34] and is produced in the United Kingdom by LGC. The third type is a pharmacogenetic test for clozapine-induced agranulocytosis [35], PGxPredict:Clozapine, marketed by PGxHealth [36]. And fourthly, a test for metabolic syndrome (PhyzioType system) [37,38] has patent applications pending by Genomas [39].

This section first describes targets of the various tests: CYP testing, clozapine response, clozapine-induced agranulocytosis, and antipsychotic-induced metabolic syndrome; then, a description of each test is given. Because CYP testing may be more widely used by clinicians and has a greater level of complexity, its description is more extensive. This article does not focus on genetic tests designed to diagnose risk for psychiatric disorders because they are not pharmacogenetic tests. A recent article has described some tests marketed, or ready to be marketed, for psychiatric diagnoses [40].

CYP testing

To introduce the practical issues involved, this CYP section reviews the cytochromes P450 2D6 (CYP2D6), 2C19 (CYP2C19), and 2C9

(CYP2C9). The current limited information on the clinical relevance of CYP tests is provided.

Cytochrome P450 2D6

CYP2D6 metabolizes several antipsychotic and antidepressant drugs [41]. CYP2D6 is highly polymorphic, meaning that more than 60 alleles and more than 130 genetic variations (a combination of SNPs and CNVs) have been described for this gene, located on chromosome 22 [41,42]. The activity level of the CYP2D6 enzyme, called the CYP2D6 phenotype, can vary widely because of different combinations of the various CYP2D6 alleles. The most important phenotype is the poor metabolizer (PM) phenotype. PMs have no CYP2D6 activity (either inactive enzymes or no enzyme) because they have two nonfunctional CYP2D6 alleles. The prevalence of PMs is approximately 7% in Caucasians and 1% to 3% in other races [14,41,43]. Also important are gene duplications that may lead to ultrarapid metabolizer (UM) phenotypes. CYP2D6 duplications were described in two families of depressive patients in Sweden who were taking tricyclic antidepressants (TCAs) and had low blood levels despite their self-reported medication adherence [44]. One family had 3 active CYP variants: one chromosome had 1 active variant and the other chromosome had a duplication of an active variant. The other family had 13 active CYP2D6 variants: one chromosome had 1 active gene copy and the other chromosome had 12 copies of an active form, called a multiplication [44]. Unfortunately, it has become clear that not all duplications or multiplications are associated with higher activity [25]. One has a duplication of an inactive allele that is associated with no activity (eg, $2 \times 0 = 0$). The Swedish subjects who metabolized TCAs at an accelerated rate were called UMs [44]. A UM can be defined as a subject who has three or more copies of an active CYP2D6 gene [25,45]. Other investigators have used the term "UM" as the equivalent of possessing a duplication but, from the pharmacologic point of view, this terminology is erroneous because some duplications can be associated with no activity or less than normal activity. The danger of making "duplication" and "UM phenotype" equivalent is not great in Caucasians in the United States because most American Caucasians who have duplications are UMs. But it is a substantial error in African Americans. More than one half of the African Americans who have duplications are not UMs; in fact, some African American subjects who have inactive duplications can be PMs [25]. The prevalence of subjects who have duplications is 1% in Sweden, up to 10% in southern Europe, and up to 29% in northern Africa and the Middle East [14,41]. The published UM prevalences may be incorrect because some articles have wrongly interpreted duplications as the equivalent of UMs. A recent comprehensive, worldwide study suggested that perhaps up to 40% in North Africa and more than 20% in some populations of Oceania are CYP2D6 UMs [46]. In a recent large study in the United States, the prevalence of CYP2D6 UMs was 1% to 2% in Caucasians and African Americans [47]. Recent studies in the United States [48] and Germany [49] suggest that multiplications are probably rare; most UMs may have a duplication of an active gene variant and a normal gene copy in the other chromosome.

Normal subjects are designated extensive metabolizers (EMs). EMs have at least one active CYP2D6 copy but less than three active copies [45]. Others have proposed that subjects who have only one active copy should be called intermediate metabolizers (IMs) [24]. A narrow definition of IM phenotype includes only those who have an activity level of greater than zero but less than one normal active CYP2D6 copy [45]; this definition selects some subjects who have less than normal activity. Some IMs are closer to PMs, whereas others may be closer to EMs. The issue of the IM phenotype is further complicated by race and drug specificity. Among East Asians (China, Japan, and nearby countries), the most frequent CYP2D6 allele is *10, an allele with lower activity than normal [50]. The average East Asian has two copies of *10/*10 and CYP2D6 activity lower than normal. However, PMs among East Asians are rare (< 1%). The interpretation of CYP2D6 activity gets even more complicated in Black Africans and African Americans, where allele *17 is frequent [51]. Traditionally, the allele was described as being associated with low activity for several CYP2D6 substrates [52]. However, *17 appears to be associated with normal activity for metabolizing risperidone [53].

Limited attempts have been made to propose personalizing dosing for psychiatric drugs. Kirchheiner and colleagues [24] attempted to personalize dosing using studies of blood levels, assuming that these medications follow linear kinetics. They proposed modifying some antipsychotic and antidepressant dosages, based on the fact that some of them are metabolized by some polymorphic CYP isoenzymes. The authors attempted to make guidelines friendlier to clinicians by focusing on clinically relevant changes, using their clinical experience with genotyping and acknowledging that not all antidepressants follow linear pharmacokinetics [14,54]. More recently, it has become clear that the concept of the therapeutic window is necessary in understanding how CYP polymorphic variation may influence personalized prescription [47]. Box 1 [13,24,47,54–67] summarizes the current status of all clinical applications of CYP2D6 testing.

CYP2C19

CYP2C19 [68] is also a polymorphic gene located on chromosome 10, with three major alleles. The most frequent allele is *1 and it has normal activity. Two alleles with no activity, *2 and *3, were initially described. The *2 allele is particularly frequent in East Asians: approximately 10% to 25% of East Asians are CYP2C19 PMs. Less than 5% of subjects from other races are CYP2C19 PMs [68]. Alleles *4 to*8 are inactive but

Box 1. Possible role of cytochrome P450 2D6 and P450 2C19 genotyping focused in psychiatry

1. *CYP2D6 genotyping and prodrugs (activated by CYP2D6)*
   Codeine
   > CYP2D6 PMs may be protected from dependence [55]/ respond with no analgesia and adverse drug reactions [56,57].
   > CYP2D6 UMs may show morphine intoxication [58,59].
   > Breast-feeding mothers should not use it [60].
   Oxycodone and hydrocodone
   > CYP2D6 UMs may show opioid intoxication [61].
   Other opioids that may be prodrugs are tramadol and dihydrocodeine [56].
   Diphenhydramine
   > CYP2D6 UMs may show paradoxic excitation [62].

2. *CYP2D6 genotyping and antipsychotics*
   Phenothiazines
   > CYP2D6 PMs should be treated with approximately one half the dose [14,24].
   Haloperidol
   > CYP2D6 PMs should be treated with lower doses [14,24].
   > It should be avoided in CYP2D6 UMs [14,24].
   Risperidone
   > CYP2D6 PMs should be treated with approximately one half the dose [14].
   > CYP2D6 PMs can be identified by therapeutic drug monitoring (TDM) [14,63].
   > (CYP2D6 UMs may need higher doses but it has not been well studied [14]).
   Aripiprazole
   > Not enough data exist to provide dose recommendations [14,47].

3. *CYP2D6 and CYP2C19 genotyping and antidepressants*
   TCAs
   > CYP2D6 PMs or CYP2C19 PMs should be treated with approximately one half the dose [14,24].
   > High doses under TDM should be considered for CYP2D6 UMs [14,24].
   > (CYP2C19 UMs may need higher doses; it has not been studied).
   Venlafaxine
   > Not enough data exist to provide dose recommendations according to CYP2D6 phenotypes [14,24,47].

Paroxetine and fluoxetine
  No clear data are available on the relevance of CYP2D6
    phenotypes [14,24,47].
Sertraline
  No clear data are available on the relevance of CYP2C19
    phenotypes [14,24].
Citalopram and escitalopram
  CYP2C19 PMs may respond better to average doses [47].
  CYP2C19 UMs may need higher doses [47,64].
Subjects intolerant to most antidepressants may be PMs for
  CYP2D6 and CYP2C19 (rare; <1% in all races). Mirtazapine
  or bupropion may be better choices [65].

4. *CYP2D6 genotyping and medication for attention deficit*
disorder
  Amphetamines
    No clear data are available on the clinical relevance of
      CYP2D6 phenotypes.
  Atomoxetine
    CYP2D6 PMs may respond better to average doses [47,66].
    CYP2D6 UMs may need higher doses but it has never been
      studied [47].

5. *CYP2C19 genotyping and benzodiazepines*
  Diazepam
    CYP2C19 PMs appear to have greater sedation with usual
      doses [67].
Most suggestions have limited information to support them other
  than pharmacokinetic science and this information changes
  rapidly because of our limited knowledge [13,24,47,54].

rare [68]. Recently, a new variant of CYP2C19 (*17) has been described that may be associated with the UM phenotype for CYP2C19 drugs [69]. The described prevalence of homozygous subjects (*17/*17) among 146 Swedes was 2.7% [69]. No studies have been published of this new allele in the population of the United States. Box 1 describes the current status of the clinical applications of CYP2C19 testing. Some extreme cases of CYP PMs are PMs for CYP2D6 and CYP2C19. They are probably rare subjects (<1% in all races) [65].

CYP2C9

The CYP2C9 gene is adjacent to that of CYP2C19 and is also polymorphic. CYP2C9 is also involved in drug metabolism of relevance to medicine (warfarin and nonsteroidal anti-inflammatory drugs). CYP2C9 represents a minor metabolic pathway for some antidepressants [70] and its polymorphisms may be important in psychiatric patients deficient for other CYP enzymatic activities [29].

CYP tests available

Two genotyping methods are reviewed in detail because they are frequently used in laboratories in the United States and, more importantly, they have peer-reviewed articles describing their characteristics. The AmpliChip CYP 450 Test [25,26] was cleared for clinical use by the FDA at the beginning of 2006; the Luminex Tag-It Mutation Detection Kit [29–31] is currently approved for research use only. A prior article [25] described other CYP genotyping methods mainly used for research purposes and the commercial laboratories in the United States providing CYP genotyping.

The European Union approved Jurilab's DrugMet Genotyping Test [71] in May 2006. However, Jurilab's Web site [71] does not currently (2008) list the test, and the investigators have seen one article using the DrugMet Genotyping Test as a confirmatory test [72]. Most of these common CYP genetic variants are easy to genotype and their characterization could be performed in clinical and research laboratories by different techniques. Alternatively, an increasing number of commercial laboratories and biotech companies offer genotyping services for polymorphisms in CYP and other metabolizing enzymes at competitive prices. The kits described, with standardized protocols and validated detection methods, should make it even easier to determine the CYP metabolizing status of patients before treatment, and their cost and sometimes complex equipment requirements should not constitute a deterrent to implementing CYP genotyping in clinical settings.

The AmpliChip CYP450 Test

The AmpliChip CYP450 Test [25,26] uses Affy metrix [1] technology. The microarray contains more than 15,000 oligonucleotide probes, allowing testing for 20 CYP2D6 alleles (*1, *2, *3, *4, *5, *6, *7, *8, *9, *10, *11, *15, *17, *19, *20, *29, *35, *36, *40, and *41), 7 CYP2D6 duplications (*1xn, *2xn, *4xn, *10xn, *17xn, *35xn, and *41xn), and 3 CYP2C19 alleles (*1, *2, and *3) [27]. Compared with traditional methods, the AmpliChip CYP450 Test has the advantage of not relying on the identification of a normal allele by default. It has wild-type and mutant probe sets. The inclusion of software using algorithms to predict the CYP2D6 and CYP2C19 phenotypes is another major advance. The initial steps of the AmpliChip CYP450 Test are similar to traditional methods and involve polymerase chain reaction amplification of selected DNA segments, followed by application of the fragmented, labeled DNA to the microarray for hybridization and staining, laser-scanning of the fluorescent hybridization intensity pattern, and then software interpretation of the genotype and phenotype [27].

The Tm Tag-It Mutation Detection Kit

The Luminex Tag-It Mutation Detection Kit [25,29–32] uses the Luminex microsphere-based universal array genotyping platform. The test was originally developed by TMBiosciences, which was acquired by Luminex in 2007 [32]. The Detection Kit for CYP2C19 detects the two most frequent CYP2C19 null alleles (*2 and *3) and five other rare null alleles (*4,*5,*6,*7,*8). It appears to be a good system for detecting PMs for CYP2C19 and CYP2D6. It identifies the wild-type CYP2D6 allele by genotyping 12 tested mutant alleles and gene arrangements associated with deletion and duplication genotypes. However, it does not include some of the CYP2D6 low-functioning alleles, has no phenotyping software, and does not specify which allele may be duplicated [25]. The lack of specification of which allele is duplicated is a serious shortcoming and complicates the assignment of phenotype [25]. The Detection Kit for CYP2C9 detects five variants (*2, *3, *4, *5, and *6).

Test of treatment efficacy

Clozapine efficacy

Twenty years ago, a classic study demonstrated that 30% of treatment-refractory patients who did not respond to other antipsychotics responded to clozapine [73]. Meta-analyses have consistently demonstrated that clozapine may be the most efficacious antipsychotic [74]. The development of a genetic test that would predict the likelihood of response to clozapine would increase the number of patients who could benefit from this drug at an earlier stage.

LGC clozapine response test

Arranz and colleagues [33] designed a system in which a combination of variants in the gene coding for 5-HT2A, 5-HT2C, H2 receptors, and the serotonin transporter 5-HTT predict clozapine response; this pharmacogenetic test generated a lot of interest and was one of the first attempts to develop a pharmacogenetic test in psychiatry. However, other investigators were not able to replicate the predictive results of the test in patients from different clinical settings [75–77]. An improvement of this test, incorporating a number of as-yet-undisclosed genetic variants, is available for the prediction of clozapine response through the United Kingdom company LGC [34].

Test of agranulocytosis secondary to clozapine treatment

Clozapine-induced agranulocytosis

Clozapine treatment is associated with risk for agranulocytosis. The use of required weekly white blood cell monitoring and a national registry in the United States has led to a decrease in agranulocytosis to less than 1% [78].

In the past, clozapine agranulocytosis was associated with HLA variants in Ashkenazi Jews [79].

PGxPredict:Clozapine test

Genaissance Pharmaceuticals, Inc. (a pharmacogenetics company) developed a genetic test to predict clozapine-induced agranulocytosis (data presented in Table 1). The presentation at a scientific meeting [35] showed that five genes (two of the HLA-complex) were associated with clozapine-induced agranulocytosis. Genaissance Pharmaceuticals, Inc. was acquired by Clinical Data (a diagnostic company) in 2005. The pharmacogenetic branch of Clinical Data (called PGxHealth) named this test PGxPredict: Clozapine, but it is not currently described on the company's Web site [36]. However, the test will not obviate the need for a monitoring test for agranulocytosis when under clozapine treatment.

Test for metabolic syndrome associated with antipsychotic treatment

Metabolic syndrome

The metabolic syndrome [80] is a combination of abdominal obesity, hyperglycemia, hyperlipidemia, and hypertension that contributes to

Table 1
Evaluation of pharmacogenetic testing in specific clinical studies in psychiatry

	Sensitivity	Specificity	Accuracy	PPV	NPV	LRPT	LRNT
The AmpliChip CYP450 Test							
CYP2D6 PM							
phenotype [26]							
ADRs of 325 R patients[a]	16%	77%	94%	0.44[b]	0.79[b]	2.7	0.89
D/C due to ADRs	9%	63%	97%	0.38[b]	0.79[b]	3.0	0.94
of 212 R patients[a]							
Luminex Tag-It Mutation	Only allelic frequency characterization [29–31]						
Detection Kit							
LGC clozapine response test[c]							
Clozapine response in	96%	38%	77%	0.76	0.82	4.4[b]	0.11[b]
200 patients [33]							
PGxPredict:Clozapine							
33 cases and	80%[d]	80%[d]					
54 controls [35]							
PhyzioType system	Genetic association discovery [37,38] only						

Abbreviations: ADRs, adverse drug reactions; D/C, discontinuation; LRNT, likelihood ratio of a negative test; LRPT, likelihood ratio of a positive test; NPV, negative predictive value; PPV, positive predictive value; R, risperidone.

  [a] The reference provides comparison with other estimations (eg, risperidone therapeutic drug monitoring).

  [b] Values estimated for this article based on formulas from reference [88].

  [c] These values correspond to the clozapine prediction test published by Arranz et al [33]. No published values exist for the modified clozapine test commercialized by LGC.

  [d] Reference [35] did not provide data on the sample used to estimate these values.

cardiovascular risk. Metabolic syndrome is much more frequent in psychiatric patients taking antipsychotics than in the general population [81,82], to the point that it is considered an epidemic [83]. Most antipsychotics (particularly some of the so-called "atypical antipsychotics," but also some of the typicals) increase the risk for obesity, probably by increasing appetite (blocking brain receptors, including H_1 and 5-HT_{2C}) [15,84,85]. Some of the atypical antipsychotics (particularly olanzapine and clozapine) also appear to interfere directly with glucose [15,84] and lipid metabolism [15,85]. It is possible that some other antipsychotics, including quetiapine and phenothiazines such as chlorpromazine, may also interfere with lipid metabolism [15,85].

Phyziotype system

Genomas [37], a personalized medicine company, has patents pending (Patent Application Publication US 2006/0234262A1) for the PhyzioType system [37,38]. The system uses an ensemble of DNA markers from several genes, coupled with a biostatistical algorithm, to predict an individual's risk for developing adverse drug reactions, including the antipsychotic-induced metabolic syndrome. The current prototype DNA microarray includes 384 SNPs from 222 genes, representing insulin resistance, glucose metabolism, energy homeostasis, adiposity, apolipoproteins and receptors, fatty acids and cholesterol metabolism, lipases and receptors, cell signaling and transcriptional regulation, growth factors, drug metabolism, blood pressure, vascular signaling, endothelial dysfunction, coagulation and fibrinolysis, vascular inflammation, cytokines, neurotransmitter systems (serotonin, dopamine, cholinergic, histamine, glutamate), and behavior (satiety) [38]. The biostatistical algorithm is based on physiogenomics, the medical application of sensitivity analysis and systems engineering. Sensitivity analysis is the study of the relationship between input and output, as determined by each system component. Physiogenomics uses genes as the components of the system [37]. The PhyzioType system in under development for use related to weight gain [37] and to the direct effects of antipsychotics on hyperlipidemia [38].

Evaluation of pharmacogenetic testing in clinical practice

Some pharmacogenetic review articles [86] insist on suggesting that the model developed by pharmaceutical companies, that of introducing a new drug into the market by sponsoring double-blind randomized trials, should be used as the ideal evidence-based model for introducing pharmacogenetic testing into the market. This approach does not appear to be reasonable from the scientific point of view because pharmacogenetic tests are not drugs, which need to be proven effective in the controlled environment of a clinical trial with randomized and placebo design; they are diagnostic tests that must be proven useful in the complex clinical environment. Feinstein and Horwitz [87] indicated 10 years ago that the evidence-based approach did not address the issue of diagnostic tests. Only recently has the evidence-based medicine approach begun considering the peculiarities of new diagnostic tests, including concepts such as pharmacological mechanism response, linkage to clinical outcome or toxicity, replication/ confirmation, and analytic validation [88]. Traditionally, the scientific properties of diagnostics have been assessed using the concepts of sensitivity (true positive rate) and specificity (true negative rate), which can be used to estimate other derived measures: accuracy, the likelihood ratio of a positive/negative test, and the likelihood ratio of positive/negative predictive value [89,90]. At first glance, defining the sensitivity and specificity of a pharmacogenetic test would seem simple. However, one can think of several levels of sensitivity and specificity: in the determination of genetic variation in the laboratory, and of genetic phenotype in the laboratory and the clinical environment [25]. These three levels of sensitivity/specificity have previously been discussed concerning the AmpliChip CYP450 Test [25]. The first level of sensitivity/specificity refers to the ability of the AmpliChip CYP450 Test to identify the mutant versus nonmutant allele distinction. The second level of sensitivity/specificity refers to the detection of each of the four CYP2D6 phenotypes [25]. The third level of sensitivity/specificity refers to the ability of a phenotype (eg, CYP2D6 PM) to make clinical predictions.

Table 1 refers to the limited published information on sensitivity/specificity in a clinical study of the pharmacogenetic tests described. This information refers to a specific sample in a specific clinical environment. These properties may vary in other samples in other clinical environments, which brings to mind the concept of generalizability, a major problem for predicting tests [91]. Only predictors that are strong and consistent are generalizable to different clinical settings. These concepts can be expressed in statistical terms but have not been sufficiently explored in the medical literature. Egmont-Petersen and colleagues [92] used the terminology of signal-to-noise ratio (coming from electrical engineering) to define the robustness of a diagnostic test. The idea is that "noise" makes the proper classification of each case (the "signal") difficult. The "noise" can come from the laboratory (eg, a problem in the technology, the interpretation of genotypes) or from the clinical environment (eg, changes in phenotype due to the effects of environmental confounders in genotypes, drug dose variability, and racial variability in genotype–phenotype relationships). The development of technologies that permit massive and generalized genetic testing should be heralded as a breakthrough but, at the same time, as a major methodological challenge, because we currently lack the statistical techniques to determine which of the thousands of genetic variations that can currently be examined may be relevant and generalizable to different clinical settings, or symptom/phenotype specific [19].

Cost effectiveness

Because the expense of health care in the United States has increased dramatically in recent years, it appears reasonable to consider the cost effectiveness of these tests [93]. A pilot study of the cost effectiveness of CYP2D6 testing [94] and a model for pharmacogenetic testing for clozapine have been published [95]. However, one needs to acknowledge that many medical advances are not cost effective. In psychiatry, the switch from typical to atypical antipsychotics has been associated with a remarkable increase in drug costs (probably by a factor of six) without reduced expenses in other types of medical care [96].

Perhaps the best laboratory test to compare with pharmacogenetic testing is a drug blood level, technically called therapeutic drug monitoring (TDM), which could be considered a phenotypic test of metabolic enzymes [97]. Almost no studies of TDM cost effectiveness exist [98], except for some studies of antibiotics. However, TDM appears to be standard clinical practice (medical insurers routinely reimburse for it) for classic anticonvulsants, theophylline, digoxin, immunosuppressants, and some psychiatric drugs [98].

Regulatory oversight

Advances in clinical genetic testing have far outpaced the regulatory framework needed to assure its safety and effectiveness. More importantly, Javitt [99] explains that the success of genetic testing depends, therefore, on the development of a coherent framework for oversight that provides adequate assurance of the safety and effectiveness of genetic tests and an equitable and stable regulatory playing field. The Secretary's Advisory Committee on Genetics, Health and Society (SACGHS), which advises the Secretary of Health and Human Services, has recently reviewed pharmacogenomic testing [100]. The committee has considered three aspects of pharmacogenomic test evaluation, including analytic validity, clinical validity and clinical utility. Analytic validity addresses accurate and reliable measurement of the genotype; clinical validity, the ability to detect or predict the associated disorder; and clinical utility, the risks and benefits of test use. In general, analytic validity is high for chip- and bead-based genomic methodologies, with sensitivity and specificity in excess of 99%. On July 26, 2007, the FDA [101] issued a draft guidance for "In Vitro Diagnostic Multivariate Index Assays (IVDMIAs)," indicating an intent to require IVDMIAs to meet premarket and postmarket device requirements under FDA regulations.

Future of pharmacogenetic testing in psychiatry

Pharmacogenetics may be moving faster in psychiatry than in other areas of medicine, with the possible exception of oncology [11]. CYP2D6 genotyping has recently become a focus of major interest in oncology because

CYP2D6 PMs may not respond to tamoxifen treatment of breast cancer [102].

The US National Institutes of Health funded the Clinical Antipsychotic Trials of Intervention Effectiveness (CATIE) study [103], which suggested that the first antipsychotic a psychiatrist prescribes for a patient may not be the best choice for that individual patient. Therefore, the future of "personalized medicine" in psychiatry, with better pharmacokinetic and pharmacodynamic genetic testing, could ultimately lead to better clinical outcomes. Studies such as CATIE may help clinical researchers change their focus from the current approach used by pharmaceutical companies, which is to try to find the best drug for the average patient. Prescription guidelines for the "average" patient may not be helpful or appropriate for the patient who has multiple comorbidities or comedications [13].

For a pharmacogenetic test to be successful in the psychiatric market, extensive clinician education will be needed [25]. Personalized medicine will require sophisticated clinicians [46] who use not only pharmacogenetic testing but environmental information (eg, comedications) and personal information (eg, gender and age) to personalize prescriptions for each patient. Health professionals have a crucial role in the future of pharmacogenetics, too. When assessing pharmacogenetic tests, health professionals need to consider the level of evidence and the cost effectiveness of pharmacogenetic testing within the context of other diagnostic tests. To compare the introduction of new pharmacogenetic tests with the introduction of a new drug into the market is not reasonable because the economic benefits and the health risks are completely different; they will be much lower in both cases for a new pharmacogenetic test. Finally, the five tests described here, the Roche AmpliChip CYP450 Test [25–28], the Luminex Tag-It Mutation Detection Kit, [29–32], the LGC clozapine response test [33,34], the PGxPredict:Clozapine [35,36], and the Genomas PhyzioType system [37–38], are the first generation of pharmacogenetic tests applied in psychiatric medicine. Technological innovations will enable various new and even spectacular advances with clinical implications, such as pharmacogenetic testing for warfarin using nanotechnology. This new test was approved by the FDA in September 2007 [104]. The advantage this technology offers is that results can be obtained in a few hours, providing busy clinicians with rapid answers [69].

Acknowledgments

The authors thank Lorraine Maw, MA, for editorial assistance.

References

[1] Fodor SP. Massively parallel genomics. Science 1997;277:393–5.
[2] Golden F, Lemonick MD. The race is over. Time 2000;3:18–23.

[3] McKusick VA. The anatomy of the human genome: a neo-vesalian basis for medicine in the 21st century. JAMA 2001;286:2289–95.

[4] Redon R, Ishikawa S, Fitch KR, et al. Global variation in copy number in the human genome. Nature 2006;444:444–54.

[5] Emery J, Hayflick S. The challenge of integrating genetic medicine into primary care. BMJ 2001;322:1027–30.

[6] Phillips KA, Veenstra DL, Oren E, et al. Potential role of pharmacogenomics in reducing adverse drug reactions: a systematic review. JAMA 2001;286:2270–9.

[7] Roses AD. Pharmacogenetics and drug development: the path to safer and more effective drugs. Nature Rev Genet 2004;5:645–56.

[8] Science. New research horizons. Science 1997;278:2039.

[9] Lertola J. Deciphering the code and what might come from it. Time 1999;8:68–9.

[10] Collins FS, McKusick VA. Implications of the human genome project for medical science. JAMA 2001;285:540–4.

[11] Cappell K, Arndt M, Carey J. Drugs get smart. Bus Week 2005;5:76–85.

[12] Wedlund PJ, de Leon J. Cytochrome P450 2D6 and antidepressant toxicity and response: what is the evidence? Clin Pharmacol Ther 2004;75:373–5.

[13] de Leon J, Armstrong SC, Cozza KL. The dosing of atypical antipsychotics. Psychosomatics 2005;46:262–73.

[14] de Leon J, Armstrong SC, Cozza KL. Clinical guidelines for psychiatrists for the use of pharmacogenetic testing for CYP450 2D6 and CYP450 2C19. Psychosomatics 2006;47:75–85.

[15] de Leon J, Diaz FJ. Planning for the optimal design of studies to personalize antipsychotic prescriptions in the post-CATIE era: the clinical and pharmacoepidemiological data suggest that pursuing the pharmacogenetics of metabolic syndrome complications (hypertension, diabetes mellitus and hyperlipidemia) may be a reasonable strategy. Schizophr Res 2007;96:185–97.

[16] Arranz MJ, Kerwin RW. Neurotransmitter-related genes and antipsychotic response: pharmacogenetics meets psychiatric treatment. Ann Med 2000;32:128–33.

[17] Arranz MJ, Munro J, Osborne S, et al. Applications of pharmacogenetics in psychiatry: personalisation of treatment. Expert Opin Pharmacother 2001;2:537–42.

[18] Arranz MJ, Collier D, Kerwin RW. Pharmacogenetics for the individualization of psychiatric treatment. Am J Pharmacogenomics 2001;1:3–10.

[19] Arranz MJ, de Leon J. Pharmacogenetics and pharmacogenomics of schizophrenia: a review of the last decade of research. Mol Psychiatry 2007;12:707–47.

[20] Ruano G. Quo vadis personalized medicine. Personalized Med 2004;1:1–7.

[21] Wang SJ, Cohen N, Katz DA, et al. Retrospective validation of genomic biomarkers—what are the questions, challenges and strategies for developing useful relationships to clinical outcomes—workshop summary. Pharmacogenomics J 2006;6:82–8.

[22] Pathway Diagnostics. Available at: http://www.pathwaydx.com/proprietary/biomarker_portfolio.php. Accessed March 23, 2008.

[23] Mayo Clinic Laboratory. Available at: http://mayomedicallaboratories.com. Accessed March 23, 2008.

[24] Kirchheiner J, Nickchen K, Bauer M, et al. Pharmacogenetics of antidepressants and antipsychotics: the contribution of allelic variations to the phenotype of drug response. Mol Psychiatry 2004;9:442–73.

[25] de Leon J. The AmpliChip CYP450 Test: personalized medicine has arrived in psychiatry. Expert Rev Mol Diagn 2006;6:277–86.

[26] de Leon J, Susce MT, Murray-Carmichael E. The AmpliChip CYP450 Genotyping Test: integrating a new clinical tool. Mol Diagn Ther 2006;10:135–51.

[27] Roche AmpliChip CYP450 Test. Available at: http://www.roche.com/home/products/prod_diag_amplichip.htm. Accessed March 23, 2008.

[28] Roche Molecular Systems, Inc. AmpliChip CYP450 Test for in vitro diagnostic use. Branchburg (NJ): Roche Molecular Systems, Inc.; 2005.

[29] Ruaño G, Makowski G, Windemuth A, et al. High carrier prevalence of deficient and null alleles of CYP2 genes in a major USA hospital: implications for personalized drug safety. Personalized Med 2006;3:131–7.

[30] Melis R, Lyon E, McMillan GA, et al. Determination of CYP2D6, CYP2C9 and CYP2C19 genotypes with Tag-It™ mutation detection assays. Expert Rev Mol Diagn 2006;6:811–20.

[31] Scott SA, Edelmann L, Kornreich R, et al. CYP2C9, CYP2C19 and CYP2D6 allele frequencies in the Ashkenazi Jewish population. Pharmacogenomics 2007;8:721–30.

[32] Luminex. Available at: http://www.luminexcorp.com/technology/xtag/index.html. Accessed March 23, 2008.

[33] Arranz MJ, Munro J, Birkett J, et al. Pharmacogenetic prediction of clozapine response. Lancet 2000;355:1615–6.

[34] LGC. Available at: http://www.lgc.co.uk/service.asp?intElement=6314. Accessed March 23, 2008.

[35] Malhotra AK, Athanasiou M, Reed CR, et al. Discovery of genetic markers associated with clozapine induced agranulocytosis. Am J Med Genet B Neuropsychiatr Genet 2005;138b:22.

[36] PGxHealth. Available at: http://www.pgxhealth.com/genetictests. Accessed March 23, 2008.

[37] Ruaño G, Goethe JW, Caley C, et al. Physiogenomic comparison of weight profiles of olanzapine- and risperidone-treated patients. Mol Psychiatry 2007;12:474–82.

[38] de Leon J, Correa JC, Ruaño G, et al. Exploring genetic variations that may be associated with the direct effects of some antipsychotics on lipid levels. Schizophr Res 2006;98:40–6.

[39] Genomas. Available at: http://www.genomas.net/. Accessed March 23, 2008.

[40] Couzin J. Gene tests for psychiatric risk polarizes psychiatry. Science 2008;319:274–7.

[41] Ingelman-Sundberg M. Genetic polymorphisms of cytochrome P450 2D6 (CYP2D6): clinical consequences, evolutionary aspects and functionary diversity. Pharmacogenomics J 2005;5:6–13.

[42] CYP450. Available at: http://www.cypalleles.ki.se. Accessed March 23, 2008.

[43] Bradford LD. CYP2D6 allele frequency in European Caucasians, Asians, Africans and their descendants. Pharmacogenomics 2002;3:229–43.

[44] Johansson I, Lundqvist E, Bertilsson L, et al. Inherited amplification of an active gene in the cytochrome P450 CYP2D locus as a cause of ultrarapid metabolism of debrisoquine. Proc Natl Acad Sci U S A 1993;90:11825–9.

[45] Chou WH, Yan FX, Robbins-Weilert DK, et al. Comparison of two CYP2D6 genotyping methods and assessments of genotype-phenotype relationships. Clin Chem 2003;49:542–51.

[46] Sistonen J, Sajantila A, Lao O, et al. CYP2D6 worldwide genetic variation shows high frequency of altered activity variants and no continental structure. Pharmacogenet Genomics 2007;17:93–101.

[47] de Leon J. The crucial role of the therapeutic window in understanding the clinical relevance of the poor versus the ultrarapid metabolizer phenotypes in subjects taking drugs metabolized by CYP2D6 and CYP2C19. J Clin Psychopharmacol 2007;27:241–5.

[48] Candiotti KA, Birnbach DJ, Lubarsky DA, et al. The impact of pharmacogenomics on postoperative nausea and vomiting: do CYP2D6 allele copy number and polymorphisms affect the success or failure of ondansetron prophylaxis? Anesthesiology 2005;102:543–9.

[49] Kirchheiner J, Schmidt H, Tzvetkov M, et al. Pharmacokinetics of codeine and its metabolite morphine in ultra-rapid metabolizers due to CYP2D6 duplication. Pharmacogenomics J 2007;7:257–65.

[50] Johansson I, Oscarson M, Yue Q-Y, et al. Genetic analysis of the Chinese cytochrome P4502D locus: characterization of variant CYP2D6 genes present in subjects with diminished capacity for debrisoquine hydroxylation. Mol Pharmacol 1994;46:452–9.

[51] Gaedigk A, Bradford LD, Marcucci KA, et al. Unique CYP2D6 activity distribution and genotype-phenotype discordance in black Americans. Clin Pharmacol Ther 2002;72:76–89.

[52] Wennerholm A, Dandara C, Sayi J, et al. The African-specific CYP2D6*17 allele encodes an enzyme with changed substrate specificity. Clin Pharmacol Ther 2002;71:77–88.

[53] Cai WM, Nikoloff DM, Pan RM, et al. CYP2D6 genetic variations in healthy adults in psychiatric African-American subjects: implications for clinical practice and genetic testing. Pharmacogenomics J 2006;6:343–50.

[54] de Leon J. Incorporating pharmacogenetics into clinical practice: reality of a new tool in psychiatry. Current issues in clinical implementation. CNS Spectr 2006;11(Suppl 3):8–12.

[55] Tyndale RF, Droll KP, Sellers EM. Genetically deficient CYP2D6 metabolism provides protection against oral opiate dependence. Pharmacogenetics 1997;7:375–9.

[56] Lotsch J, Starke C, Liefhold J, et al. Genetic predictors of the clinical response to opioid analgesics: clinical utility and future perspectives. Clin Pharmacokinet 2004;43:983–1013.

[57] Susce MT, Murray-Carmichael E, de Leon J. Response to hydrocodone, codeine and oxycodone in a CYP2D6 poor metabolizer. Prog Neuropsychopharmacol Biol Psychiatry 2006;30:1356–8.

[58] Dalen P, Frengell C, Dahl ML, et al. Quick onset of severe abdominal pain after codeine in an ultrarapid metabolizer of debrisoquine. Ther Drug Monit 1997;19:543–4.

[59] Gasche Y, Daali Y, Fathi M, et al. Codeine intoxication associated with ultrarapid CYP2D6 metabolism. N Engl J Med 2004;351:2827–31.

[60] Koren G, Cairns J, Chitayat D, et al. Pharmacogenetics of morphine poisoning in a breastfed neonate of a codeine-prescribed mother. Lancet 2006;368:704.

[61] de Leon J, Dinsmore L, Wedlund PJ. Adverse drug reactions to oxycodone and hydrocodone in CYP2D6 ultrarapid metabolizers. J Clin Psychopharmacol 2003;23:420–1 [letter].

[62] de Leon J, Nikoloff DM. Paradoxical excitation on diphenhydramine may be associated with being a CYP2D6 ultrarapid metabolizer: three case reports. CNS Spectr 2008;13:133–5.

[63] de Leon J, Susce MT, Pan RM, et al. A study of genetic (CYP2D6 and ABCB1) and environmental (drug inhibitors and inducers) variables that may influence plasma risperidone levels. Pharmacopsychiatry 2007;40:93–102.

[64] Rudberg I, Mohebi B, Hermann M, et al. Impact of the ultrarapid CYP2C19*17 allele on serum concentration of escitalopram in psychiatric patients. Clin Pharmacol Ther 2008;83:322–7.

[65] Johnson M, Markham-Abedi C, Susce MT, et al. A poor metabolizer for both cytochrome P450 2D6 and 2C19 (CYP2D6 and CYP2C19): a case report on antidepressant treatment. CNS Spectr 2006;11:757–60.

[66] Wernicke JF, Kratochvil CJ. Safety profile of atomoxetine in the treatment of children and adolescents with ADHD. J Clin Psychiatry 2002;63(Suppl 12):50–5.

[67] Inomata S, Nagashima A, Itagaki F, et al. CYP2C19 genotype affects diazepam pharmacokinetics and emergence from general anesthesia. Clin Pharmacol Ther 2005;78:647–55.

[68] Wedlund PJ. The CYP2C19 enzyme polymorphism. Pharmacology 2000;6:174–85.

[69] Sim SC, Risinger C, Dahl ML, et al. A common novel CYP2C19 gene variant causes ultrarapid drug metabolism relevant for the drug response to proton pump inhibitors and antidepressants. Clin Pharmacol Ther 2006;79:103–13.

[70] Black JL 3rd, O'Kane DJ, Mrazek DA. The impact of CYP allelic variation on antidepressant metabolism: a review. Expert Opin Drug Metab Toxicol 2007;3:21–31.

[71] Jurilab. Available at: http://www.jurilab.com. Accessed March 23, 2008.

[72] Lee HK, Lewis LD, Tsongalis GJ, et al. Validation of a CYP2D6 genotyping panel on the NanoChip Molecular Biology Workstation. Clin Chem 2007;53:823–8.

[73] Kane J, Honigfield G, Singer J, et al. Clozapine for the treatment resistant schizophrenic: a double blind comparison with chlorpromazine (Clozaril Collaborative Study). Arch Gen Psychiatry 1998;45:789–96.

[74] Davis JM, Chen N, Glick ID. A meta-analysis of the efficacy of second-generation antipsychotics. Arch Gen Psychiatry 2003;60:553–64.

[75] Schumacher J, Schulze TG, Wienker TF, et al. Pharmacogenetics of the clozapine response. Lancet 2000;356:506–7.

[76] Arranz MJ, Munro J, Osborne S, et al. Difficulties in replication of results. Lancet 2000;356:1359–60.

[77] Arranz MJ, Munro J, Sham P, et al. Meta-analysis of studies on genetic variation in 5-HT2A receptors and clozapine response. Schizophr Res 1998;32:93–9.

[78] Alvir JM, Lieberman JA, Safferman AZ, et al. Clozapine-induced agranulocytosis: incidence and risk factors in the United States. N Engl J Med 1993;329:162–7.

[79] Lieberman JA, Yunis J, Egea E, et al. HLA-B38, DR4, DQw3 and clozapine-induced agranulocytosis in Jewish patients with schizophrenia. Arch Gen Psychiatry 1990;47:945–8.

[80] Ford ES, Giles WH, Dietz WH. Prevalence of the metabolic syndrome among US adults. JAMA 2002;287:356–9.

[81] Susce MT, Villanueva N, Diaz FJ, et al. Obesity and associated complications in patients with severe mental illnesses: a cross-sectional survey. J Clin Psychiatry 2005;66:167–73.

[82] McEvoy JP, Meyer JM, Goff DC, et al. Prevalence of the metabolic syndrome in patients with schizophrenia: baseline results from the Clinical Antipsychotic Trials of Intervention Effectiveness (CATIE) schizophrenia trial and comparison with national estimates from NHANES III. Schizophr Res 2005;80:19–32.

[83] Reist C, Mintz J, Albers LJ, et al. Second-generation antipsychotic exposure and metabolic-related disorders in patients with schizophrenia: an observational pharmacoepidemiology study from 1988 to 2002. J Clin Psychopharmacol 2007;27:46–51.

[84] Newcomer JW, Haupt DW. The metabolic effects of antipsychotic medications. Can J Psychiatry 2006;51:480–91.

[85] Meyer JM, Koro CE. The effects of antipsychotic therapy on serum lipids: a comprehensive review. Schizophr Res 2004;70:1–17.

[86] Grossman I. Routine pharmacogenetic testing in clinical practice: dream or reality? Pharmacogenomics 2007;8:1449–59.

[87] Feinstein AR, Horwitz RI. Problems in the "evidence" of "evidence-based medicine". Am J Med 1997;103:529–35.

[88] Altar CA, Amakye D, Bounos D, et al. A prototypical process for creating evidentiary standards for biomarkers and diagnostics. Clin Pharmacol Ther 2008;83:368–71.

[89] Greenhalgh T. Papers that report diagnostic or screening tests. Br Med J 1997;315:540–3.

[90] Deeks JJ. Systematic reviews of evaluations of diagnostic and screening tests. Br Med J 2001;323:157–62.

[91] Justice AC, Covinsky KE, Berlin JA. Assessing the generalizability of prognostic information. Ann Intern Med 1999;130:515–24.

[92] Egmont-Petersen M, Talmon JL, Hasman A. Robustness metrics for measuring the influence of additive noise on the performance of statistical classifiers. Int J Med Inform 1997;46:103–12.

[93] Wedlund PJ, de Leon J. Pharmacogenetic testing: the cost factor. Pharmacogenomics J 2001;1:171–4.

[94] Chou WH, Yan FX, de Leon J, et al. Extension of a pilot study: impact from the cytochrome P450 2D6 polymorphism on outcomes and costs associated with severe mental illness. J Clin Psychopharmacol 2000;20:246–51.

[95] Perlis RH, Ganz DA, Avorn J, et al. Pharmacogenetic testing in the clinical management of schizophrenia: a decision-analytic model. J Clin Psychopharmacol 2005;25:427–34.

[96] Duggan M. Do new prescription drugs pay for themselves? The case of second-generation antipsychotics. J Health Econ 2005;24:1–31.

[97] Ensom MH, Chang TK, Patel P. Pharmacogenetics: the therapeutic drug monitoring of the future? Clin Pharmacokinet 2001;40:783–802.

[98] Touw DJ, Neef C, Thomson AH, et al. Cost-effectiveness of therapeutic drug monitoring: a systematic review. Ther Drug Monit 2005;27:10–7.

[99] Javitt GH. In search of a coherent framework: options for FDA oversight of genetic tests. Food Drug Law J 2007;62:617–52.

[100] The Secretary's Advisory Committee on Genetics. Health and Society (SACGHS) has recently reviewed pharmacogenomic testing. Available at: http://www4.od.nih.gov/oba/sacghs/reports/CR_report.pdf. Accessed March 23, 2008.

[101] FDA. In vitro diagnostic multivariate index assays (IVDMIAs). Available at: http://www. fda.gov/cdrh/oivd/guidance/1610.pdf. Accessed March 23, 2008.

[102] Beverage JN, Sissung TM, Sion AM, et al. CYP2D6 polymorphisms and the impact on tamoxifen therapy. J Pharm Sci 2007;96:2224–31.

[103] Lieberman JA, Stroup TS, McEvoy JP, et al. Effectiveness of antipsychotic drugs in patients with chronic schizophrenia. N Engl J Med 2005;353:1209–23.

[104] Nanosphere announces FDA clearance of second molecular diagnostics assay. Available at: http://ir.nanosphere.us/phoenix.zhtml?c=214748&;p=irol-newsArticle&ID=1075929 &highlight=. Accessed March 23, 2008.

CLINICS IN
LABORATORY
MEDICINE

ELSEVIER
SAUNDERS

Clin Lab Med 28 (2008) 619–626

Pharmacogenetics-Guided Dose Modifications of Antidepressants

Angela Seeringer, MD, Julia Kirchheiner, MD*

Institute of Pharmacology of Natural Products and Clinical Pharmacology, University of Ulm, Helmholtzstrasse 20, 89081 Ulm, Germany

Rationale behind the development of pharmacogenetic diagnostics: genotype-based dosing

Individual dosing of drugs in general is performed according to the (1) expected individual drug exposure, (2) individual risk for adverse drug effects or, rarely, (3) expected drug efficacy. Genetic variability in drug metabolism as reflected in differences in clearance, half-life, and maximal plasma concentrations is highly replicable and can be considered for genotype-based dose adjustments. These dose adjustments can be calculated according to the principles of bioequivalence while considering special circumstances, including linearity of pharmacokinetics, activity of metabolites, and dose range of the underlying studies. Methods for extracting dose adjustments from genotype-specific pharmacokinetic data have been developed and published elsewhere [1–3].

Genetic differences in pharmacokinetic parameters such as oral clearances could be overcome through adjusting the drug dose. In Fig. 1, a scheme for adjusting individual dosages according to the drug metabolizing genotypes predicting ultrahigh, high, intermediate and slow metabolic activity is depicted, and can be derived from the differences in plasma concentration courses. These theoretic dose adjustments make sense for the drug therapies in which a similar plasma concentration time course also leads to similar clinical effects. In antidepressant drug therapy, however, plasma concentrations correlate poorly with clinical efficacy, and therefore genotype-based dose adjustments will mostly address the risk for adverse drug effects.

Fig. 2 shows the differential doses of antidepressants due to polymorphisms of *CYP2D6* given for the poor (PM), intermediate (IM), extensive

* Corresponding author.

E-mail address: julia.kirchheiner@uni-ulm.de (J. Kirchheiner).

0272-2712/08/$ - see front matter © 2008 Elsevier Inc. All rights reserved.
doi:10.1016/j.cll.2008.05.006   *labmed.theclinics.com*

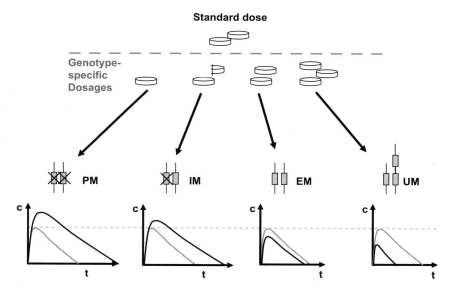

Fig. 1. Principle of calculation of genotype-based dose adjustments based on differences in pharmacokinetic parameters, such as clearance and area under the curve. The theoretic dosages for genetic subgroups of poor (PMs), intermediate (IMs), extensive (EMs), and ultrarapid metabolizers (UMs) are depicted as schematic genotype-specific dosages to obtain equal plasma concentration time courses. C, concentration; T, time. (*From* Kirchheiner J, Nickchen K, Bauer M, et al. Pharmacogenetics of antidepressants and antipsychotics: the contribution of allelic variations to the phenotype of drug response. Mol Psychiatry 2004;9(5):442–73; with permission.)

(EM), and ultrarapid (UM) metabolizer genotypes. The figure shows that the amount of dose adaptation varies among substrates, and that clinically relevant differences in dosages exist for some antidepressants, whereas others are only slightly influenced by the CYP2D6 polymorphism.

Limitations of pharmacogenetic dose adjustments

When calculating quantitative dose adjustments from genotype-specific pharmacokinetic data, several points have to be considered. Metabolites with their own pharmacologic activity often exist, eliciting therapeutic activity and possibly causing adverse effects. Thus, if considerable concentrations of active metabolites exist in plasma, they should be acknowledged in the dosing adjustments either through summarizing the whole active drug compound or deciding to make no dose adjustment and recommending a change in drug choice (if metabolites are generated that have potential for adverse drug effects).

The sample size and power of the existing data must be large enough to derive dose adjustments. Data on carriers of homozygous variations should at least be available. Furthermore, the dose range of the studies from which

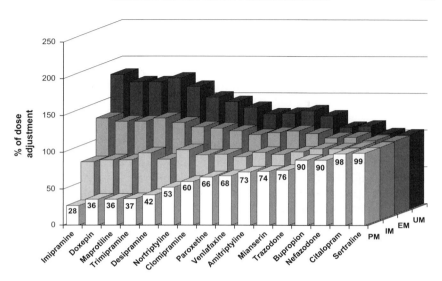

Fig. 2. *CYP2D6* genotype dependent quantitative changes in pharmacokinetics of antidepressant drugs expressed as percent dose adaptations. CYP2D6 PM (*white*), IM (*gray*), EM (*dark gray*), UM (*black*). Dose adaptations were calculated as described in [1]. Dose adaptations are based on an average dose of 100% and are aimed for the Caucasian population. Data from studies in Asiatic or African or other populations were not incorporated because PM data are lacking. (*From* Kirchheiner J, Nickchen K, Bauer M, et al. Pharmacogenetics of antidepressants and antipsychotics: the contribution of allelic variations to the phenotype of drug response. Mol Psychiatry 2004;9(5):442–73; with permission.)

dose adjustments are derived should be in the clinical range, although this does not often occur because many studies are performed on healthy volunteers using lower drug doses. However, dose recommendations cannot be extrapolated automatically to the dose range used in patients.

Comedication must be considered. Different genotypes lead to different consequences from interacting substances. For example, changes in enzyme activity from substances that are inducers or inhibitors of an enzyme cannot occur in genetic poor metabolizers. In contrast, EMs or UMs can convert to phenotypic poor metabolizers through strong enzyme inhibitors. Thus, genotype-based dose adjustments must be weighed against changes in phenotype caused by comedication.

Prospective validation of genotype-based dose adjustments is necessary, and several studies are now comparing therapy using pharmacogenetic diagnostics with standard therapy in a randomized controlled fashion.

Clinical implications of pharmacogenetic testing in psychiatry

In psychiatry and geriatrics, 52% of psychiatric, 49% of psychogeriatric, and 46% of geriatric patients use at least one drug metabolized by CYP2D6, whereof 62% are classified as antidepressants or antipsychotics [4]. Therefore, CYP2D6 has a special relevance in psychiatry and in the treatment of depression and schizophrenia.

Another highly polymorphic enzyme, CYP2C19, also participates in biotransformation of some tricyclic antidepressants, including amitriptyline, imipramine, and clomipramine [5]. Thus, genotyping for CYP2D6 and CYP2C19 might help optimize antidepressant drug treatment, especially for the treatment with tricyclic antidepressants [6].

Although genotyping for individualized dosing demands quick and on-site available pharmacogenetic diagnostic tools, psychiatric practice typically performs genotyping after an adverse drug reaction has occurred or when patients experience no response to various antidepressant drugs. Most often, pharmacogenetic diagnostics are applied together with therapeutic drug monitoring, particularly in patients who develop extensively high or low drug concentrations at standard dosages.

Although huge differences in drug concentrations are observed from prospective studies in individuals who have different genotypes, these monogenetic differences decrease in clinical relevance because of many other sources of variability [7]. In addition, dosages are empirically adjusted by the physicians or patients themselves because of individual patient needs, and differences in the empirically chosen drug dosage are frequently observed when comparing carriers of different genotypes [8–13].

Despite this decrease in effect size of a genetic factor in clinical practice compared with the standardized study conditions, there are situations where it certainly would make sense to know an individual's genotype before the start of a drug therapy. These situations include drug therapies with a narrow therapeutic index, drugs for which direct outcome or response parameters cannot be assessed, and drug therapies, where a loss in drug efficacy can be dangerous for the patient, for example when using anticancer drugs. When looking at these typical situations, genotype-based dosing seems relevant for antidepressant drug therapy because of a high risk for adverse drug effects and a lack of parameters predicting drug response (approximately 30% of all patients who have depression do not respond sufficiently to the first antidepressant drug [14]). The use of pharmacogenetic variants as biomarkers for antidepressant drug response, however, is restricted because of the poor plasma concentration–response relationship and the empiric dose modifications in patients who have special metabolizer genotypes.

Impact of *CYP2D6* and *CYP2C19* polymorphisms on pharmacokinetics and outcome of antidepressant drugs

The group of tricyclic antidepressants undergoes biotransformation in the liver, with CYP2D6 catalyzing hydroxylation or demethylation reactions [15]. PMs of CYP2D6 have largely (50% or more) decreased clearances for amitriptyline, clomipramine, desipramine, imipramine, nortriptyline, doxepin, and trimipramine [1]. Thus, individuals for whom tricyclic antidepressants are prescribed could benefit from *CYP2D6* genotyping, if the dose is subsequently adjusted for the group of PMs and UMs identified through testing.

Some selective serotonin reuptake inhibitors (SSRIs), such as fluoxetine, fluvoxamine, and paroxetine, are potent inhibitors of CYP2D6 activity. Therefore, multiple dosing causes autoinhibition of CYP2D6 and conversion from extensive to slow metabolizer phenotype and from ultrafast to extensive metabolism [16,17]. In the case of fluvoxamine, differences in areas under the curve (AUCs) were described after single doses [18,19], whereas multiple doses result in similar AUCs in PMs and EMs, indicating a strong inhibitory effect on CYP2D6 in EMs [20].

Although paroxetine is also a CYP2D6 inhibitor, twofold higher AUCs of the drug were observed in CYP2D6 PMs than in EMs after multiple doses [21]. In another study, one UM carrying at least three functional *CYP2D6* gene copies had undetectable drug concentrations [17]. In contrast, no influences of *CYP2D6* polymorphisms on pharmacokinetic parameters of sertraline and citalopram have been observed. Moclobemide, sertraline, and citalopram are metabolized by CYP2C19 and CYP2D6, and differences in AUCs in CYP2C19 PMs were approximately twofold (moclobemide and citalopram) or less (sertraline) [22–24]. However, these genotypic influences detected in pharmacokinetic studies in healthy volunteers did not translate into differences in drug response or adverse drug reactions in citalopram treatment in the largest clinical sample of patients treated with citalopram (Star*D study) [25]. Thus, within the group of SSRIs, CYP inhibition poses a problem for drug interaction, but growing evidence shows that assessment of cytochrome P450 polymorphisms may not be clinically useful for guiding SSRI therapy.

For mirtazapine, *CYP2D6* genotype was shown to have a significant influence on the variability in the plasma concentration; however, when comparing UMs with EMs, the magnitude of concentration differences was only moderate [1]. CYP2D6 is responsible for transforming venlafaxine to the equipotent O-desmethyl-venlafaxine [26–29]. A higher risk for cardiotoxic events and other adverse drug effects might exist in PMs [30], because cases of severe arrhythmia have been reported in four patients treated with venlafaxine who were all CYP2D6 PMs [31]. By contrast the *CYP2D6* polymorphism seems to have no major influence on metabolism of duloxetine, nefazodone, moclobemide, reboxetine, and trazodone.

Several studies have shown that differences in pharmacokinetic parameters caused by genetic polymorphisms impact therapeutic outcome and risk for adverse drug reactions with antidepressant use. In a German study evaluating the effect of *CYP2D6* genotype on adverse effects and nonresponse during treatment with CYP2D6-dependent antidepressants, PMs and UMs were significantly overrepresented compared with the control population in the patients experiencing adverse drug reactions (fourfold) and nonresponders (fivefold), respectively [32].

However, Grasmader and colleagues [33] did not find any influence of *CYP2D6* and *CYP2C19* genotype on antidepressant drug response, although the incidence of relevant side effects tended to be higher in PMs of CYP2D6. Furthermore, a prospective 1-year clinical study of 100 psychiatric inpatients suggested a trend toward longer hospital stays and higher treatment costs for UMs and PMs of CYP2D6 [34].

Thus, for treatment with antidepressants, considerable evidence shows that *CYP2D6* polymorphisms, and to a lesser extent those of *CYP2C19*, affect the pharmacokinetics of several antidepressants, and possibly therapeutic outcome and adverse drug events. The usefulness of genotyping procedures in patients who have depression, however, has not been confirmed in prospective clinical trials; therefore, this approach is currently limited to a few hospitals and some patients who have adverse or lacking therapeutic effects.

References

[1] Kirchheiner J, Nickchen K, Bauer M, et al. Pharmacogenetics of antidepressants and antipsychotics: the contribution of allelic variations to the phenotype of drug response. Mol Psychiatry 2004;9(5):442–73.

[2] Kirchheiner J, Brosen K, Dahl ML, et al. CYP2D6 and CYP2C19 genotype-based dose recommendations for antidepressants: a first step towards subpopulation-specific dosages. Acta Psychiatr Scand 2001;104(3):173–92.

[3] McLeod HL, Siva C. The thiopurine S-methyltransferase gene locus—implications for clinical pharmacogenomics. Pharmacogenomics 2002;3(1):89–98.

[4] Mulder H, Heerdink ER, van Iersel EE, et al. Prevalence of patients using drugs metabolized by cytochrome P450 2D6 in different populations: a cross-sectional study. Ann Pharmacother 2007;41(3):408–13.

[5] Brøsen K, Gram LF. Clinical significance of the sparteine/debrisoquine oxidation polymorphism. Eur J Clin Pharmacol 1989;36(6):537–47.

[6] Steimer W, Zopf K, von Amelunxen S, et al. Amitriptyline or not, that is the question: pharmacogenetic testing of CYP2D6 and CYP2C19 identifies patients with low or high risk for side effects in amitriptyline therapy. Clin Chem 2005;51(2):376–85.

[7] Brockmoller J, Kirchheiner J, Schmider J, et al. The impact of the CYP2D6 polymorphism on haloperidol pharmacokinetics and on the outcome of haloperidol treatment. Clin Pharmacol Ther 2002;72(4):438–52.

[8] Borgiani P, Ciccacci C, Forte V, et al. Allelic variants in the CYP2C9 and VKORC1 loci and interindividual variability in the anticoagulant dose effect of warfarin in Italians. Pharmacogenomics 2007;8(11):1545–50.

[9] Kimura R, Miyashita K, Kokubo Y, et al. Genotypes of vitamin K epoxide reductase, gamma-glutamyl carboxylase, and cytochrome P450 2C9 as determinants of daily warfarin dose in Japanese patients. Thromb Res 2007;120(2):181–6.

[10] Chern HD, Ueng TH, Fu YP, et al. CYP2C9 polymorphism and warfarin sensitivity in Taiwan Chinese. Clin Chim Acta 2006;367(1–2):108–13.

[11] Sconce EA, Khan TI, Wynne HA, et al. The impact of CYP2C9 and VKORC1 genetic polymorphism and patient characteristics upon warfarin dose requirements: proposal for a new dosing regimen. Blood 2005;106(7):2329–33.

[12] Hillman MA, Wilke RA, Caldwell MD, et al. Relative impact of covariates in prescribing warfarin according to CYP2C9 genotype. Pharmacogenetics 2004;14(8):539–47.

[13] Kamali F, Khan TI, King BP, et al. Contribution of age, body size, and CYP2C9 genotype to anticoagulant response to warfarin. Clin Pharmacol Ther 2004;75(3):204–12.

[14] Bauer M, Whybrow PC, Angst J, et al. World Federation of Societies of Biological Psychiatry (WFSBP) Guidelines for Biological Treatment of Unipolar Depressive Disorders, Part 1: acute and continuation treatment of major depressive disorder. World J Biol Psychiatry 2002;3(1):5–43.

[15] Baumann P, Jonzier Perey M, Koeb L, et al. Amitriptyline pharmacokinetics and clinical response: II. Metabolic polymorphism assessed by hydroxylation of debrisoquine and mephenytoin. Int Clin Psychopharmacol 1986;1(2):102–12.

[16] Laine K, Tybring G, Hartter S, et al. Inhibition of cytochrome P4502D6 activity with paroxetine normalizes the ultrarapid metabolizer phenotype as measured by nortriptyline pharmacokinetics and the debrisoquin test. Clin Pharmacol Ther 2001;70(4):327–35.

[17] Lam YW, Gaedigk A, Ereshefsky L, et al. CYP2D6 inhibition by selective serotonin reuptake inhibitors: analysis of achievable steady-state plasma concentrations and the effect of ultrarapid metabolism at CYP2D6. Pharmacotherapy 2002;22(8):1001–6.

[18] Carrillo JA, Dahl ML, Svensson JO, et al. Disposition of fluvoxamine in humans is determined by the polymorphic CYP2D6 and also by the CYP1A2 activity. Clin Pharmacol Ther 1996;60(2):183–90.

[19] Spigset O, Granberg K, Hagg S, et al. Relationship between fluvoxamine pharmacokinetics and CYP2D6/CYP2C19 phenotype polymorphisms. Eur J Clin Pharmacol 1997;52(2): 129–33.

[20] Spigset O, Granberg K, Hagg S, et al. Non-linear fluvoxamine disposition. Br J Clin Pharmacol 1998;45(3):257–63.

[21] Sindrup SH, Brøsen K, Gram LF, et al. The relationship between paroxetine and the sparteine oxidation polymorphism. Clin Pharmacol Ther 1992;51(3):278–87.

[22] Gram LF, Guentert TW, Grange S, et al. Moclobemide, a substrate of CYP2C19 and an inhibitor of CYP2C19, CYP2D6, and CYP1A2: a panel study. Clin Pharmacol Ther 1995; 57(6):670–7.

[23] Wang JH, Liu ZQ, Wang W, et al. Pharmacokinetics of sertraline in relation to genetic polymorphism of CYP2C19. Clin Pharmacol Ther 2001;70(1):42–7.

[24] Sindrup SH, Brøsen K, Hansen MG, et al. Pharmacokinetics of citalopram in relation to the sparteine and the mephenytoin oxidation polymorphisms. Ther Drug Monit 1993;15(1): 11–7.

[25] Peters EJ, Slager SL, Kraft JB, et al. Pharmacokinetic genes do not influence response or tolerance to citalopram in the STAR*D sample. PLoS ONE 2008;3(4):e1872.

[26] Fukuda T, Yamamoto I, Nishida Y, et al. Effect of the CYP2D6*10 genotype on venlafaxine pharmacokinetics in healthy adult volunteers. Br J Clin Pharmacol 1999;47(4):450–3.

[27] Fukuda T, Nishida Y, Zhou Q, et al. The impact of the CYP2D6 and CYP2C19 genotypes on venlafaxine pharmacokinetics in a Japanese population. Eur J Clin Pharmacol 2000;56:175–80.

[28] Otton SV, Ball SE, Cheung SW, et al. Venlafaxine oxidation in vitro is catalysed by CYP2D6. Br J Clin Pharmacol 1996;41(2):149–56.

[29] Veefkind AH, Haffmans PM, Hoencamp E. Venlafaxine serum levels and CYP2D6 genotype. Ther Drug Monit 2000;22(2):202–8.

[30] Shams ME, Arneth B, Hiemke C, et al. CYP2D6 polymorphism and clinical effect of the antidepressant venlafaxine. J Clin Pharm Ther 2006;31(5):493–502.

[31] Lessard E, Yessine M, Hamelin B, et al. Influence of CYP2D6 activity on the disposition and cardiovascular toxicity of the antidepressant agent venlafaxine in humans. Pharmacogenetics 1999;9:435–43.

[32] Rau T, Wohlleben G, Wuttke H, et al. CYP2D6 genotype: impact on adverse effects and nonresponse during treatment with antidepressants-a pilot study. Clin Pharmacol Ther 2004;75(5):386–93.

626   SEERINGER & KIRCHHEINER

[33] Grasmader K, Verwohlt PL, Rietschel M, et al. Impact of polymorphisms of cytochrome-P450 isoenzymes 2C9, 2C19 and 2D6 on plasma concentrations and clinical effects of antidepressants in a naturalistic clinical setting. Eur J Clin Pharmacol 2004;60(5):329–36.
[34] Kawanishi C, Lundgren S, Agren H, et al. Increased incidence of CYP2D6 gene duplication in patients with persistent mood disorders: ultrarapid metabolism of antidepressants as a cause of nonresponse. A pilot study. Eur J Clin Pharmacol 2004;59(11):803–7.

ELSEVIER
SAUNDERS

CLINICS IN
LABORATORY
MEDICINE

Clin Lab Med 28 (2008) 627–643

Pharmacogenetic Testing in Schizophrenia and Posttraumatic Stress Disorder

Bronwyn Ramey-Hartung, PhD[a],[*],
Rifaat S. El-Mallakh, MD[b],
Kristen K. Reynolds, PhD[a],[c]

[a]PGXL Laboratories, Louisville, KY 40202, USA
[b]Mood Disorders Research Program, Department of Psychiatry and Behavioral Sciences, University of Louisville School of Medicine, Louisville, KY 40202, USA
[c]Department of Pathology and Laboratory Medicine, University of Louisville School of Medicine, Louisville, KY 40202, USA

Many psychiatric medications have a narrow therapeutic range, below which patients may see no therapeutic effects and above which patients begin to experience adverse reactions. Standard pharmacological therapy begins with a first-line drug. If treatment fails or the patient experiences adverse effects over a period of time, physicians often switch patients to a second drug. If this therapy also fails, physicians then often choose a drug from a different class. This can lead, for many patients, to a months-long ordeal of pharmacological trial and error. For psychiatric patients, such delays in achieving therapeutic status can be particularly troubling, leading to lost time at work, increased costs, and increased risk of experiencing adverse side effects, all of which can exacerbate a patient's psychiatric condition. These problems also lead to decreased compliance among patients who are unwilling to tolerate the side effects and the long wait for therapeutic benefit. Genotyping patients prior to beginning psychiatric pharmacological therapy can serve to inform practitioners as to each patient's likelihood of therapeutic response and their relative risk of experiencing toxicity and other adverse side effects from certain drugs. Such information could arm physicians with the knowledge they need to make appropriate drug and dosing decisions and avoid the lengthy trial-and-error process with which they are faced today.

* Corresponding author. PGXL Laboratories, 201 E. Jefferson Street, Suite 309, Louisville, KY 40202, USA

E-mail address: bronwyn.ramey@pgxlab.com (B. Ramey-Hartung).

0272-2712/08/$ - see front matter © 2008 Elsevier Inc. All rights reserved.
doi:10.1016/j.cll.2008.08.004 *labmed.theclinics.com*

Schizophrenia

Schizophrenia is a severe psychiatric illness that manifests with waxing and waning psychotic symptoms, such as hallucinations or delusions, or a significant thought disorder. These symptoms are usually superimposed over more persistent negative symptoms (eg, amotivation, social indifference, reduced self-care, and cognitive deficits). Pharmacologic treatment focuses on control of the dramatic psychotic symptoms and is of minimal benefit for the more chronic negative symptoms. All effective antipsychotic agents exhibit significant blockade of the dopamine D2 receptor (DRD2) [1]. First-generation antipsychotics (FGAs), such as the phenothiazines (eg, chlorpromazine, fluphenazine, perphenazine) or the butyropherones (eg, haloperidol), are primary D2 antagonists. Newer second-generation antipsychotics (SGAs) also block the D2 receptor and additionally block the serotonin receptor 2A ($5HT_{2A}$). This action is believed to reduce dopamine release in the striatum and to increase its release in the prefrontal cortex [1]. Consequently, SGAs provide equal and possibly superior efficacy for both the positive symptoms of psychosis [2] and the negative symptoms [3] with fewer adverse effects on the central nervous system [4].

The major drawback of FGAs is their propensity to induce motor system abnormalities. Acutely, these manifest as parkinsonism and akathisia [5]. Chronic exposure leads to tardive dyskinesia, which manifests with choreaform movements of perioral, facial, and upper body muscles, and, more rarely, of the trunk and lower limbs [6]. Dystonias and a perioral tremor known as rabbit syndrome may also occur [6]. Both acute parkinsonism and chronic tardive dyskinesia can be disabling and disfiguring. Parkinsonism develops in over 60% of schizophrenic subjects receiving an FGA [7], and the rates may be higher when mood-disturbed patients take FGAs [8]. SGAs have lower rates of extrapyramidal symptoms, which may approach the rates seen with placebo [8,9]. Tardive dyskinesia may develop in 15% to 30% of schizophrenic patients receiving FGAs, and is more common in patients with central nervous system injury; chronic medical conditions, such as diabetes; and in the elderly [6]. The experience of drug-induced parkinsonism predicts subsequent development of tardive dyskinesia [10].

The adverse effect profile of SGAs is different from that of FGAs. Some SGAs appear to increase appetite with consequent weight increase, increase serum cholesterol and triglycerides, and reduce glucose regulation [11,12]. The US Food and Drug Administration (FDA) has inserted a class warning regarding glucose control for all SGAs. Additionally, many of these agents are heavily dependent on cytochrome P450 metabolism, so that coadministration with agents that either stimulate or inhibit P450 enzymes may result in either an increase in adverse effects or a reduction in efficacy.

These adverse effects play an important role in the tolerability of and adherence to antipsychotic medications. Nearly 75% of schizophrenic patients discontinue their antipsychotic medication within 18 months of treatment [13]. Noncompliance is one of the major correlates of increased morbidity in schizophrenia [14].

Posttraumatic stress disorder

Awareness of posttraumatic stress disorder (PTSD) is growing among the general public because of the recent focus in the popular media on the incidence of the disorder among returning Iraq War veterans. In reality, PTSD affects more civilians than soldiers in the United States, although PTSD rates are higher in combat soldiers, affecting 14% to 18% of those exposed to combat [15,16], while only 7.8% of the American population is affected [17]. Only a fraction of people exposed to severe trauma develop PTSD, which suggests that predisposing factors may be important in defining risk. A recent study of Iraq War combat veterans found that injury is one such factor. In the study population, only 9.1% of uninjured veterans developed PTSD, while 43.9% of those having loss of consciousness developed PTSD [15]. There are also several lines of evidence that now suggest a genetic vulnerability to the development of PTSD.

Mice in which the serotonin transporter (5-HTT) has been knocked out are much more susceptible to lasting anxiety symptoms after exposure to predator stress [18]. In humans, a natural variant of the serotonin transporter carries a 44–base-pair (bp) deletion in the promoter region (thus termed *short*) that reduces both transcription of the gene and translation of its messenger RNA, yielding an overall 50% reduction in expression of the serotonin transporter protein [19–22]. This short form variant is also strongly associated with PTSD [23]. A study of Hurricane Katrina victims found that those who possessed the short form and had poor social support were 4.5 times more likely to develop PTSD and depression than those who did not have these predisposing factors [24]. This important role of the serotonin transporter might explain why serotoninergic antidepressants are important in the treatment of PTSD (see discussion below).

Major depression

Major depression is a common psychiatric illness associated with significant morbidity [25]. The illness is usually episodic and manifests with a depressed mood; reduced energy; changes in appetite, sleep, and concentration; and psychological symptoms, such as reduced self-esteem and suicidal ideation. As many as 10% of people may experience a depressive episode at some point in their lives, with women more commonly affected than men. Despite its frequency, more than half of the patients with this illness remain untreated [26]. Unfortunately, the longer the duration of the illness, the poorer the outcome, with an increased rate of recurrence [27]. Effective treatment for depression has been available for nearly two generations. Older medications, the tricyclic antidepressants and

monoamine oxidase inhibitors, largely have been replaced with selective serotonin reuptake inhibitors (SSRIs) and serotonin-norepinephrine reuptake
inhibitors (SNRIs), which have better safety profiles. While the newer antidepressants are generally safer than the older drugs, they still carry a large
adverse-effect liability. These include somatic adverse effects, such as sexual
dysfunction and gastrointestinal disturbance, and central nervous system
adverse effects, such as agitation and insomnia. Additionally, many of the
SSRIs are potent P450 enzyme inhibitors, which put patients at increased
risk for drug-drug interactions.

Tricyclic and tetracyclic antidepressants are named according to their
chemical structure. These agents are believed to have their antidepressant
action by inhibition of reuptake of serotonin and norepinephrine from the
synaptic gap [28,29]. Tri- and tetracyclic medications are effective in relieving symptoms of depression and anxiety, and may even provide more effective relief than that provided by SSRIs. However, because of their associated
risk of adverse effects, tri- and tetracyclic medications are rarely used in first-
line therapy [30–34]. Adverse effects associated with the tri- and tetracyclic
medications include sexual dysfunction and gastrointestinal upset, as well as
a host of anticholinergic effects, including dry mouth, constipation, urinary
retention, and blood-pressure dysregulation. The most worrisome adverse
effect of these medications is the slowing of cardiac conduction and subsequent risk of ventricular arrhythmia, particularly in overdose [35,36]. This
property is particularly problematic since these medications are frequently
given to people with suicidal ideation.

SSRIs and SNRIs are generally safer in overdosage in comparison to the
tri- and tetracyclics, but can still be fatal [37]. Adverse effects, which appear
to be related to their serotonergic action, are common with these drugs and
may impact compliance [38,39]. For instance, erectile dysfunction in men
and anorgasmia in both men and women affect the majority of patients
receiving SSRI/SNRI antidepressants [40,41]. While erectile dysfunction is
treatable with the addition of sildenafil, anorgasmia is more difficult to
manage [42,43]. Furthermore, antidepressant discontinuation is also
problematic: A discontinuation syndrome has been described that
complicates antidepressant use [44]. One of the most problematic adverse
effects of all antidepressants is the propensity toward manic induction or
destabilization of the course of bipolar illness in both type I and II bipolar
patients [45].

The FDA has mandated a label warning that antidepressant use can
increase suicidal ideation in adolescents and young adults receiving these
agents [46]. This was based on a review of 4582 pediatric participants in
24 antidepressant trials. There were no completed suicides in any of these
patients, but suicidal ideation and suicidal behaviors were nearly twice as
common among recipients of antidepressants as those receiving placebo
[46]. The FDA decision, which has been the focus of significant controversy,
is likely a factor in the recent decline in antidepressant use among youths

[47]. Interestingly, this decline in antidepressant use appears to have been associated with an increase in suicide rates [48].

Pharmacogenetics in treatment response

Some psychiatric medications have a narrow therapeutic range, below which patients may see no therapeutic effects and above which patients begin to experience adverse reactions. Antipsychotic-induced adverse reactions can include extrapyramidal syndromes, such as parkinsonism and tardive dyskinesia, the latter of which can sometimes be irreversible. The antipsychotic clozapine, an important SGA used in patients who are nonresponsive to other antipsychotics, can also lead to agranulocytosis, a rare but potentially fatal condition associated with HLA variants [49–51]. Because of their effects on appetite (via the serotonin system) and lipid and glucose metabolism, antipsychotics may also cause substantial weight gain and diabetes. Patients receiving antipsychotic therapy with any antipsychotic are at risk of developing neuroleptic malignant syndrome, which manifests as hyperthermia and is accompanied by muscle stiffness, rhabdomyolysis, and autonomic disturbances, which may be fatal [52]. Those antipsychotics with strong binding affinity for the dopamine receptors are strongly associated with increases in prolactin levels, putting patients at risk of experiencing lactation and reduced libido [53,54]. Antipsychotic-induced adverse reactions can include a host of gastrointestinal problems, sleep disturbances, and sexual dysfunction, as well as extrapyramidal symptoms, including tardive dyskinesia. Not only can these adverse effects pose a severe health risk to patients, they also contribute substantially to noncompliance.

CYP450 metabolic variants

Variation in the cytochrome P450 (CYP) system, CYP2D6 and CYP2C19 in particular, can lead to aberrant drug levels and increase patients' risk of experiencing adverse drug reactions. In the case of psychiatric medications, the therapeutic dosing of up to 60% of antidepressants and antipsychotics is largely dependent on CYP2D6 and CYP2C19. Some antipsychotic drugs, however, are metabolized by alternate metabolic pathways, making the application of CYP pharmacogenetic diagnostics to these drugs more difficult [55,56]. Kirchheiner and colleagues, [57,58] in this publication and elsewhere, have recommended using CYP2D6, CYP2C19, and CYP2C9 genotyping to make therapeutic dosing adjustments for patients receiving antidepressant and antipsychotic therapy. In general, patients who, because of their genetic characteristics, are classified as CYP poor metabolizers are more likely to develop increased blood concentrations of the drug and potentially experience adverse effects at common dosages, while ultra-rapid metabolizers are more likely to exhibit subtherapeutic drug concentrations and experience inadequate efficacy [57,58]. Additional consideration must be given in cases where patients are taking concomitant medications. Patients with chronic or terminal illnesses are often prescribed medications for depression/anxiety in addition to other drugs, such as opioids for chronic pain, tamoxifen for breast cancer, and beta-blockers for arrhythmia or hypertension. Patients may experience compounded toxicities in cases where co-administered drugs are metabolized via the same enzyme. When a patient's metabolic status is altered either by genetic variation or drug-gene interaction, the toxicity risks of either or both drugs may be increased, or the given drugs may have reduced therapeutic benefit.

While metabolic phenotyping based on CYP genotype testing may significantly improve psychiatric therapy by reducing the risk of toxicity and improving compliance (and thereby treatment efficacy), pharmacokinetics tell only half the story. In fact, controversy still remains regarding the influence of metabolizer status on the effectiveness of psychiatric medications [59]. Some of the apparent disagreement can be accounted for by the variable quality or breadth of the studies thus far published, but may in other cases be better explained by the unrecognized influence of genetic variables affecting the pharmacodynamics of psychiatric medications.

Receptor variants

Variations in drug receptors play an important role in determining patients' therapeutic and adverse responses. The quality of information provided by pharmacogenetics is therefore only fully realized when pharmacodynamic factors are considered in concert with pharmacokinetics (Table 1, Fig. 1).

Dopamine D_2 receptor

All antipsychotic drugs (both FGAs and SGAs) function in whole or in part via DRD2 blockade, while the SGAs additionally interact with multiple receptors, including D3 and D4, and serotonin receptors [60,61]. The differential receptor targeting and affinity of the FGAs and SGAs is the basis for their different clinical effects: FGAs, which primarily target dopamine, provide effective relief of positive symptoms but have poor effectiveness on negative symptoms, and are commonly associated with extrapyramidal symptoms [60]; however, SGAs, with their multiple targets and decreased affinity for the dopamine receptors, relieve both positive and negative symptoms, and are associated with a lower risk of extrapyramidal symptoms [62]. Conversely, SGAs carry increased risk of adverse metabolic effects. The relative effectiveness of a given antipsychotic drug is mediated by its dopamine antagonism as determined by the relative binding affinity for DRD2.

Genotypic variants of DRD2 have been associated with varying response to antipsychotics. Presence of the C nucleotide insertion at position -141 of the DRD2 promoter is associated with decreased gene expression in vivo and in vitro [63,64] (although one study found contradictory results [65]). This insertion variant does not appear to impact ultimate antipsychotic

Table 1
Pharmacokinetic and pharmacodynamic gene targets for psychotropic medications

Gene	Alleles	Drug classes affected	Mechanism	Clinical consequences
CYP2D6	*3 *4 *5 (gene deletion) *6 *7 and others	SSRIs SNRIs TCAs FGAs SGAs	Nonfunctional CYP2D6 enzyme	Decreased drug clearance, increased drug accumulation and exposure; increased risk of ADRs Associated with extrapyramidal symptoms, weight gain, cardiac arrhythmia, neuroleptic malignant syndrome
CYP2C19	*2 *3	TCAs some SSRIs SNRIs some FGAs SGAs	Nonfunctional CYP2C19 enzyme	Decreased drug clearance; increased drug accumulation and exposure; increased risk of ADRs
DRD2	Taq1A +/-	FGAs SGAs SSRIs	1A+ associated with decreased striatal DRD2 density and decreased receptor binding potential	Increased risk of PTSD following trauma; increased psychopathology scores; improved response to antipsychotics and SSRIs; increased risk of extrapyramidal symptoms with antipsychotics
	-141 C Ins/Del	FGAs SGAs	Unclear	-141 C Del associated with swifter therapeutic response
	-241A > G	FGAs SGAs	Unclear	-241G associated with improved response
5-HTT	5-HTTLPR l(long)/s(short)	SSRIs	S (short) form associated with decreased expression of 5-HTT	S form associated with increased risk of ADRs and increased time to achieve efficacy on SSRIs; may benefit from non-SSRI antidepressants Increased risk of PTSD following trauma

Abbreviations: ADR, adverse drug reaction; TCA, tricyclic antidepressant.

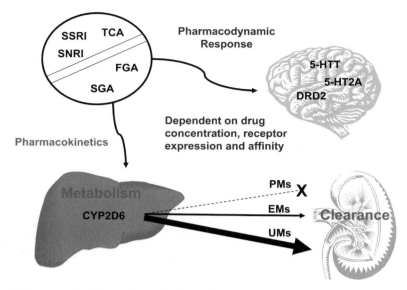

Fig. 1. Therapeutic efficacy of psychiatric medications depends on the interaction between pharmacokinetic (PK) and pharmacodynamic (PD) drug profiles. The therapeutic (PD) response to a given drug is dictated by drug occupancy of the target protein. The target number, the target affinity, and the consistency with which the drug can be concentrated on the target together mediate the interaction. The balance between drug accumulation rate (based on dosage) and clearance rate (based on metabolism) determines drug concentration. Pharmacogenetic variants in a PD pathway affect the concentration dependency of the target by altering protein affinity or expression, while variants in a metabolic PK pathway alter clearance rate, drug half-life, and concentration at the target. TCA, tricyclic antidepressant.

response [66–68]. However, Lencz and colleagues [69] found that the carriers of this variant showed a significantly longer time to respond. The investigators suggest that the decreased striatal receptor density in -141 C deletion carriers allow more efficient antipsychotic blockade for a swifter therapeutic effect. The group also found a positive association between patient response and the presence of the -241A > G variant, but the mechanism and effect of this variant on DRD2 expression and response to SGAs are unclear [69].

More consistent results have been obtained in studies examining the DRD2 Taq1A locus, so defined by a restriction fragment length polymorphism located near exon 8 in the 3′ intron of the DRD2 gene. This variant is significantly associated with changes in receptor density. The 1A+ allele has 30% to 40% frequency in Caucasians [70–72] and has been associated with decreased DRD2 density and decreased receptor dopamine binding potential [64]. DRD2 Taq1A polymorphism has implications in schizophrenia and in PTSD and major depression. In schizophrenia, Taq1A+ is consistently associated with a better response to antipsychotic therapies, although the benefit seems limited to positive, not negative, symptoms

[68,70,73–76]. While these studies were all preliminary and use rather small, ethnically homogenous (largely Japanese) samples, the consistency of the trend is encouraging and indicates a need for much larger studies.

In studies of Vietnam War veterans, the DRD2 Taq1A allele was found to be far more prevalent in combat veterans who developed PTSD (60%) than in those who did not (5%), and is associated with greater psychopathology scores in untreated PTSD patients [71,77]. A similar positive trend is found between DRD2 Taq1A and response to treatment with SSRIs, specifically paroxetine [71].

The positive effects of DRD2 Taq1A on treatment response is somewhat tempered by a significant trend toward an association with a higher (up to 2.4-fold) incidence of extrapyramidal symptoms in patients receiving antipsychotics, a trend that has been identified in European, but not Japanese, subjects [78–80]. These results create a compelling argument for the use of DRD2 Taq1A genotyping to inform drug choice in naïve schizophrenic and PTSD/depressive patients, particularly if such testing is performed in combination with CYP450 - please replace all with this revision to avoid "P" redundancy genotyping, which could inform both drug choice and dosing [79].

Serotonin transporter (5-HTT)

The serotonin transporter mediates the active reuptake of serotonin from the synaptic gap. SSRI therapies inhibit the action of the serotonin transporters and thereby indirectly lead to greater synaptic serotonin concentrations. It is this increase in synaptic serotonin that is thought to be ultimately responsible for the antidepressive response. The promoter region of 5-HTT contains GC-rich repeat elements, numbered 1 through 16, each made up of about 20 nucleotides [19]. A polymorphic 44-bp deletion within repeats 6 through 8 was discovered to negatively affect transcription [19]. The alleles are defined as the l (long) allele and the s (short) allele, with the l allele yielding more than two-fold greater transcription levels (and, thus, greater protein levels) than the s allele [19,81]. Greater 5-HTT expression by the l allele is thought to result in lower base-line levels of synaptic serotonin. Possession of the s allele increases the risk of developing depression or PTSD following adversity [23,24,82].

The l allele occurs at a frequency of 20% to 26% in Asian populations and about 53% to 55% in Caucasians [83–86]. In Caucasians and Chinese, the l/l genotype has been associated with a significantly better and faster SSRI response, while the s/s allele is associated with poor response [83,84,87–97]. In two studies in Japanese and Korean patients, one found that neither the l nor s allele had an effect on treatment response; the other observed only a slight improved response among s allele carriers [98,99]. The l allele has been associated with improved response to paroxetine, fluoxetine, sertraline, and tricyclic antidepressants in depressed patients, while the s allele has been associated with both poorer response and greater incidence of side effects, including induction of mania in bipolar patients [93,98,100–102].

It is thought that l/l individuals, in whom 5-HTT expression is greatest, experience swifter and better relief from SSRI therapies because of the greater number of targets available for inhibition by the drug. Individuals with the s/s genotype, in whom expression of 5-HTT is at low levels, have too few targets available for inhibition by SSRI therapies. These individuals also have high synaptic serotonin levels, and may be maximally down-regulated both pre- and post-synaptically, making them less amenable to SSRI modulation.

Serotonin receptor (5-HT2A)

While 5-HTT modulates synaptic serotonin reuptake back into the presynaptic neuron, the serotonin receptor (5-HT2A) partially modulates neuronal response to serotonin at the postsynaptic neuron. Two polymorphisms, which are in absolute linkage disequilibrium, have been described: 102T > C is in a noncoding region and is silent, while -1438A > G is in the promoter region [103–105]. Several studies have found a positive association between these variants and SSRI and clozapine response. One of these was a large National Institutes of Health study, the Sequenced Treatment Alternatives for Depression, in which patients were prospectively phenotyped [106]. SGAs, such as clozapine, target 5-HT2A in addition to DRD2, so variants in 5-HT2A may also have implications in schizophrenia therapy [104]. The mechanistic linkage between the 5-HT2A polymorphisms and phenotype are unclear because 102T > C is silent, and the effect of -1438G > A promoter polymorphism on receptor density has not been demonstrated. Another polymorphism, His452Tyr, has been defined and found to be associated with poor response to clozapine, but the effect was small and, again, the mechanism for the effect is unknown [104,107,108].

The future of pharmacogenetics in psychiatric practice

Genotyping for variants in metabolic enzymes, such as CYP2D6 and CYP2C19, could provide insight into a patient's ability to metabolize many psychiatric medications, including the antidepressants and antipsychotics, and thus indicate that patient's potential risk of experiencing toxicity. Information regarding that patient's receptor genotypes, such as the dopamine receptor and serotonin transporter, could provide insight as to the likelihood of a given drug's effectiveness and risk of adverse side effects. The data supporting the association between other receptor polymorphisms, such as the serotonin receptor, with drug effectiveness and the risk of adverse side effects are not yet robust enough to build well-defined clinical indications for their use as pharmacogenetic diagnostics. The data for metabolic genotyping, however, are quite robust, making metabolic genotyping suitable for immediate use in the clinical setting. As discussed above, the additional use of DRD2 Taq1A genotyping could be used to further inform drug choice for both antidepressants and antipsychotics. Again, more research, including larger study populations and more tightly controlled and narrowly defined study procedures, is required before such testing could be justified for general application.

Although large-scale prospective clinical studies are required to fully appreciate the degree to which certain pharmacogenetic tests can facilitate improved safety and efficacy of psychiatric pharmacotherapy, several pharmacogenetic tests are ready to be put into practice. Among these are the assays for metabolic variants in *CYP2D6* and *CYP2C19*, and for the receptor variants in *DRD2* and *5-HTT*. When used in concert, clinicians could be armed with sufficient information to understand the risks of toxicity and the likelihood of therapeutic benefit in the use of many common psychiatric medications (see Fig. 1). Such knowledge can facilitate proper drug choice and dosing at the initiation of therapy, as clinical strategies can be tailored to the individual patient. Such practices have the potential to save time and money, reduce patients' risk of experiencing side effects, and encourage compliance.

There are two major hurdles to entry of pharmacogenetics into wide use among the psychiatric community. The first is a lack of sufficient large-scale, long-term studies and data to support quantitative understanding of the links between various genotypes and their effects on individual therapeutic dosages: One author suggested that a study to understand the impact of CYP2D6 on therapeutic outcomes and cost benefits would require a year-long study of 2000 naïve, newly diagnosed patients [109]. The second hurdle is a lack of awareness. Many psychiatric offices and clinics conduct routine therapeutic drug monitoring for certain drugs (lithium, for example), but do not do so for most drugs. These practices may also be generally unaware of the availability of pharmacogenetic testing, of the quality and utility of the information to be obtained from pharmacogenetic testing, and of the minimally intrusive manner by which patient samples may be obtained.

In the future, we anticipate that comprehensive psychiatric pharmacogenetic profiles will be used at the initiation of psychiatric therapy to guide drug choice and dosing estimation, and throughout a patient's course as a real-time aid in patient monitoring and ongoing guidance for therapy management.

References

[1] Di Pietro NC, Seamans JK. Dopamine and serotonin interactions in the prefrontal cortex: insights on antipsychotic drugs and their mechanism of action. Pharmacopsychiatry 2007; 40(Suppl 1):S27–33.

[2] Davis JM, Chen N, Glick ID. A meta-analysis of the efficacy of second-generation antipsychotics. Arch Gen Psychiatry 2003;60(6):553–64.

[3] Möller HJ. Management of the negative symptoms of schizophrenia: new treatment options. CNS Drugs 2003;17(11):793–823.

[4] Leucht S, Pitschel-Walz G, Abraham D, et al. Efficacy and extrapyramidal side-effects of the new antipsychotics olanzapine, quetiapine, risperidone, and sertindole compared to conventional antipsychotics and placebo. A meta-analysis of randomized controlled trials. Schizophr Res 1999;35(1):51–68.

[5] Elliott KJ, Lewis S, El-Mallakh RS, et al. The role of parkinsonism and antiparkinsonian therapy in the subsequent development of tardive dyskinesia. Ann Clin Psychiatry 1994;6:197–203.

[6] Khot V, Wyatt RJ. Not all that moves is tardive dyskinesia. Am J Psychiatry 1991;148(5): 661–6.

[7] Janno S, Holi M, Tuisku K, et al. Prevalence of neuroleptic-induced movement disorders in chronic schizophrenia inpatients. Am J Psychiatry 2004;161(1):160–3.

[8] Cavazzoni PA, Berg PH, Kryzhanovskaya LA, et al. Comparison of treatment-emergent extrapyramidal symptoms in patients with bipolar mania or schizophrenia during olanzapine clinical trials. J Clin Psychiatry 2006;67(1):107–13.

[9] Nasrallah HA, Brecher M, Paulsson B. Placebo-level incidence of extrapyramidal symptoms (EPS) with quetiapine in controlled studies of patients with bipolar mania. Bipolar Disord 2006;8(5 Pt 1):467–74.

[10] Sachdev P. Early extrapyramidal side-effects as risk factors for later tardive dyskinesia: a prospective study. Aust N Z J Psychiatry 2004;38(6):445–9.

[11] Meyer JM, Davis VG, Goff DC, et al. Change in metabolic syndrome parameters with antipsychotic treatment in the CATIE Schizophrenia trial: prospective data from phase 1. Schizophr Res 2008 [Feb 5, Epub ahead of print].

[12] Perez-Iglesias R, Crespo-Facorro B, Amado JA, et al. A 12-week randomized clinical trial to evaluate metabolic changes in drug-naive, first-episode psychosis patients treated with haloperidol, olanzapine, or risperidone. J Clin Psychiatry 2007;68(11):1733–40.

[13] Lieberman JA, Stroup TS, McEvoy JP, et al. Clinical Antipsychotic Trials of Intervention Effectiveness (CATIE) investigators. Effectiveness of antipsychotic drugs in patients with chronic schizophrenia. N Engl J Med 2005;353(12):1209–23.

[14] Leucht S, Heres S. Epidemiology, clinical consequences, and psychosocial treatment of nonadherence in schizophrenia. J Clin Psychiatry 2006;67(Suppl 5):3–8.

[15] Hoge CW, McGurk D, Thomas JL, et al. Mild traumatic brain injury in U.S. soldiers returning from Iraq. N Engl J Med 2008;358(5):453–63.

[16] Frueh BC, Grubaugh AL, Acierno R, et al. Age differences in posttraumatic stress disorder, psychiatric disorders, and healthcare service use among veterans in Veterans Affairs primary care clinics. Am J Geriatr Psychiatry 2007;15(8):660–72.

[17] Kessler RC, Sonnega A, Bromet E, et al. Posttraumatic stress disorder in the National Comorbidity Survey. Arch Gen Psychiatry 1995;52(12):1048–60.

[18] Adamec R, Burton P, Blundell J, et al. Vulnerability to mild predator stress in serotonin transporter knockout mice. Behav Brain Res 2006;170(1):126–40.

[19] Heils A, Teufel A, Petri S, et al. Allelic variation of human serotonin transporter gene expression. J Neurochem 1996;66(6):2621–4.

[20] Lesch KP, Bengel D, Heils A, et al. Association of anxiety-related traits with a polymorphism in the serotonin transporter gene regulatory region. Science 1996;274:1527–31.

[21] Bradley SL, Dodelzon K, Sandhu HK, et al. Relationship of serotonin transporter gene polymorphisms and haplotypes to mRNA transcription. Am J Med Genet B Neuropsychiatr Genet 2005;136(1):58–61.

[22] Philibert RA, Sandhu H, Hollenbeck N, et al. The relationship of 5HTT (SLC6A4) methylation and genotype on mRNA expression and liability to major depression and alcohol dependence in subjects from the Iowa adoption studies. Am J Med Genet B Neuropsychiatr Genet 2007 [Epub ahead of print].

[23] Lee HJ, Lee MS, Kang RH, et al. Influence of the serotonin transporter promoter gene polymorphism on susceptibility to posttraumatic stress disorder. Depress Anxiety 2005; 21:135–9.

[24] Kilpatrick DG, Koenen KC, Ruggiero KJ, et al. The serotonin transporter genotype and social support and moderation of posttraumatic stress disorder and depression in hurricane-exposed adults. Am J Psychiatry 2007;164(11):1693–9.

[25] Kessler RC, Akiskal HS, Ames M, et al. Prevalence and effects of mood disorders on work performance in a nationally representative sample of U.S. workers. Am J Psychiatry 2006; 163(9):1561–8.

[26] Parikh SV, Lesage AD, Kennedy SH, et al. Depression in Ontario: under-treatment and factors related to antidepressant use. J Affect Disord 1999;52(1–3):67–76.

[27] Altamura AC, Dell'Osso B, Mundo E, et al. Duration of untreated illness in major depressive disorder: a naturalistic study. Int J Clin Pract 2007;61(10):1697–700.

[28] Lahti RA, Maickel RP. The tricyclic antidepressants—inhibition of norepinephrine uptake as related to potentiation of norepinephrine and clinical efficacy. Biochem Pharmacol 1971; 20(2):482–6.

[29] Sangdee C, Franz DN. Enhancement of central norepinephrine and 5-hydroxytryptamine transmission by tricyclic antidepressants. A comparison. Psychopharmacology (Berl) 1979; 62(1):9–16.

[30] Machado M, Iskedjian M, Ruiz I, et al. Remission, dropouts, and adverse drug reaction rates in major depressive disorder: a meta-analysis of head-to-head trials. Curr Med Res Opin 2006;22(9):1825–37.

[31] Arroll B, Macgillivray S, Ogston S, et al. Efficacy and tolerability of tricyclic antidepressants and SSRIs compared with placebo for treatment of depression in primary care: a meta-analysis. Ann Fam Med 2005;3(5):449–56.

[32] Zhang W, Davidson JR. Post-traumatic stress disorder: an evaluation of existing pharmacotherapies and new strategies. Expert Opin Pharmacother 2007;8(12):1861–70.

[33] Bakker A, van Balkom AJ, Spinhoven P. SSRIs vs. TCAs in the treatment of panic disorder: a meta-analysis. Acta Psychiatr Scand 2002;106(3):163–7.

[34] Rickels K, Rynn M. Pharmacotherapy of generalized anxiety disorder. J Clin Psychiatry 2002;63(Suppl 14):9–16.

[35] Roose SP, Glassman AH, Giardina EG, et al. Tricyclic antidepressants in depressed patients with cardiac conduction disease. Arch Gen Psychiatry 1987;44(3):273–5.

[36] Glassman AH. Cardiovascular effects of tricyclic antidepressants. Annu Rev Med 1984;35: 503–11.

[37] Flanagan RJ. Fatal toxicity of drugs used in psychiatry. Hum Psychopharmacol 2008; 23(Suppl 1):43–51.

[38] Sullivan PW, Valuck R, Saseen J, et al. A comparison of the direct costs and cost effectiveness of serotonin reuptake inhibitors and associated adverse drug reactions. CNS Drugs 2004;18(13):911–32.

[39] Goethe JW, Woolley SB, Cardoni AA, et al. Selective serotonin reuptake inhibitor discontinuation: side effects and other factors that influence medication adherence. J Clin Psychopharmacol 2007;27(5):451–8.

[40] Rosen RC, Marin H. Prevalence of antidepressant-associated erectile dysfunction. J Clin Psychiatry 2003;64(Suppl 10):5–10.

[41] Labbate LA, Grimes JB, Arana GW. Serotonin reuptake antidepressant effects on sexual function in patients with anxiety disorders. Biol Psychiatry 1998;43(12):904–7.

[42] Fava M, Nurnberg HG, Seidman SN, et al. Efficacy and safety of sildenafil in men with serotonergic antidepressant-associated erectile dysfunction: results from a randomized, double-blind, placebo-controlled trial. J Clin Psychiatry 2006;67(2):240–6.

[43] Nurnberg HG, Hensley PL, Gelenberg AJ, et al. Treatment of antidepressant-associated sexual dysfunction with sildenafil: a randomized controlled trial. JAMA 2003;289:56–64.

[44] van Geffen EC, Hugtenburg JG, Heerdink ER, et al. Discontinuation symptoms in users of selective serotonin reuptake inhibitors in clinical practice: tapering versus abrupt discontinuation. Eur J Clin Pharmacol 2005;61(4):303–7.

[45] El-Mallakh RS, Karippot A. Chronic depression in bipolar disorder. Am J Psychiatry 2006; 163:1137–341.

[46] Pfeffer CR. The FDA pediatric advisories and changes in diagnosis and treatment of pediatric depression. Am J Psychiatry 2007;164(6):843–6.

[47] Olfson M, Marcus SC, Druss BG. Effects of Food and Drug Administration warnings on antidepressant use in a national sample. Arch Gen Psychiatry 2008;65(1):94–101.

[48] Gibbons RD, Brown CH, Hur K, et al. Early evidence on the effects of regulators' suicidality warnings on SSRI prescriptions and suicide in children and adolescents. Am J Psychiatry 2007;164(9):1356–63.

[49] Dettling M, Cascorbi I, Roots I, et al. Genetic determinants of clozapine-induced agranulocytosis: recent results of HLA subtyping in a non-Jewish Caucasian sample. Arch Gen Psychiatry 2001;58(1):93–4.

[50] Lieberman JA, Yuni J, Egea E, et al. HLA-B38, DR4, DQw3 and clozapine-induced agranulocytosis in Jewish patients with schizophrenia. Arch Gen Psychiatry 1990;47(10):945–8.

[51] Yunis JJ, Corzo D, Salazar M, et al. HLA associations in clozapine-induced agranulocytosis. Blood 1995;86(3):1177–83.

[52] Pope HG, Keck PE, McElroy SL. Frequency and presentation of neuroleptic malignant syndrome in a large psychiatric hospital. Am J Psychiatry 1986;143:1227–33.

[53] David SR, Taylor CC, Kinon BJ, et al. The effects of olanzapine, risperidone, and haloperidol on plasma prolactin levels in patients with schizophrenia. Clin Ther 2000;22(9): 1085–96.

[54] Haddad PM, Wieck A. Antipsychotic-induced hyperprolactinaemia: mechanisms, clinical features and management. Drugs 2004;64(20):2291–314.

[55] van der Weide J, Hinrichs JW. The influence of cytochrome P450 pharmacogenetics on disposition of common antidepressant and antipsychotic medications. Clin Biochem Rev 2006;27:17–25.

[56] Arranz MJ, de Leon J. Pharmacogenetics and pharmacogenomics of schizophrenia: a review of last decade of research. Mol Psychiatry 2007;12(8):707–47.

[57] Kirchheiner J, Nickchen K, Bauer M, et al. Pharmacogenetics of antidepressants and antipsychotics: the contribution of allelic variations to the phenotype of drug response. Mol Psychiatry 2004;9(5):442–73.

[58] Kirchheiner J, Fuhr U, Brockmöller J. Pharmacogenetics-based therapeutic recommendations—ready for clinical practice? Nat Rev Drug Discov 2005;4(8):639–47.

[59] Evaluation of Genomic Applications in Practice and Prevention (EGAPP) Working Group. Recommendations from the EGAPP working group: testing for cytochrome P450 polymorphisms in adults with nonpsychotic depresion treated with selective serotonin reuptake inhibitors. Genet Med 2007;9(12):819–25.

[60] Freedman R. Schizophrenia. N Engl J Med 2003;349(18):1738–49.

[61] Miyamoto S, Duncan GE, Marx CE, et al. Treatments for schizophrenia: a critical review of pharmacology and mechanisms of action of antipsychotic drugs. Mol Psychiatry 2005; 10(1):79–104.

[62] Haro JM, Salvador-Carulla L. The SOHO (Schizophrenia Outpatient Health Outcome) study: implications for the treatment of schizophrenia. CNS Drugs 2006;20(4):293–301.

[63] Arinami T, Gao M, Hamaguchi H, et al. A functional polymorphism in the promoter region of the dopamine D2 receptor gene is associated with schizophrenia. Hum Mol Genet 1997;6(4):577–82.

[64] Jönsson EG, Nothen MM, Neidt H, et al. Polymorphisms in the dopamine D2 receptor gene and their relationships to striatal dopamine receptor density of healthy volunteers. Mol Psychiatry 1999;4(3):290–6.

[65] Pohjalainen R, Någren K, Syvälahti EK, et al. The dopamine D2 receptor 5′-flanking variant, -141 C Ins/Del, is not associated with reduced dopamine D2 receptor density in vivo. Pharmacogenetics 1999;9(4):505–9.

[66] Ohara K, Nagai M, Tani K, et al. Functional polymorphism of -141 C Ins/Del in the dopamine D2 receptor gene promoter and schizophrenia. Psychiatry Res 1998;81(2): 117–23.

[67] Mihara K, Kondo T, Suzuki A, et al. No relationship between -141 C Ins/Del polymorphism in the promoter region of dopamine D2 receptor and extrapyramidal adverse effects of selective dopamine D2 antagonists in schizophrenic patients: a preliminary study. Psychiatry Res 2001;101(1):33–8.

[68] Suzuki A, Kondo T, Mihara K, et al. The -141C Ins/Del polymorphism in the dopamine D2 receptor gene promoter region is associated with anxiolytic and antidepressive effects during treatment with dopamine antagonists in schizophrenic patients. Pharmacogenetics 2001;11(6):545–50.

[69] Lencz T, Robinson DG, Xu K, et al. DRD2 promoter region variation as a predictor of sustained response to antipsychotic medication in first-episode schizophrenia patients. Am J Psychiatry 2006;163(3):529–31.

[70] Schäfer M, Rujescu D, Giegling I, et al. Association of short-term response to Haloperidol treatment with a polymorphism in the dopamine D2 receptor gene. Am J Psychiatry 2001; 158:802–4.

[71] Lawford BR, Young RM, Noble EP, et al. D2 dopamine receptor gene polymorphism: paroxetine and social functioning in posttraumatic stress disorder. Eur Neuropsychopharmacol 2003;13:313–20.

[72] Young RM, Lawford BR, Barnes M, et al. Prolactin levels in antipsychotic treatment of patients with schizophrenia carrying the DRD2*A1 allele. Br J Psychiatry 2004;185: 147–51.

[73] Wong AH, Buckle CE, van Tol HH. Polymorphisms in dopamine receptors: What do they tell us? Eur J Pharmacol 2000;410:183–203.

[74] Suzuki A, Mihara K, Kondo T, et al. The relationship between dopamine D2 receptor polymorphism at the Taq1A locus and therapeutic response to nemonapride, a selective dopamine antagonist, in schizophrenic patients. Pharmacogenetics 2000;10(4):335–41.

[75] Kondo T, Mihara K, Suzuki A, et al. Combination of dopamine D2 receptor gene polymorphisms as a possible predictor of treatment-resistance to dopamine antagonists in schizophrenic patients. Prog NeuroPsychopharmacol Biol Psychiatry 2003;27:921–6.

[76] Yamanouchi Y, Iwata N, Suzuki T, et al. Effect of DRD2, 5-HT2A and COMT genes on antipsychotic response to risperidone. Pharmacogenomics J 2003;3:356–61.

[77] Comings DE, Muhlenan D, Gysin R. Dopamine D2 receptor (DRD2) gene and susceptibility to posttraumatic stress disorder: a study and replication. Biol Psychiatry 1996;40: 368–72.

[78] Güzey C, Scordo MG, Spina E, et al. Antipsychotic-induced extrapyramidal symptoms in patients with schizophrenia: associations with dopamine and serotonin receptor and transporter polymorphisms. Eur J Clin Pharmacol 2007;63(3):233–41.

[79] Hedenmalm K, Güzey C, Dahl M-L, et al. Risk factors for extrapyramidal symptoms during treatment with selective serotonin reuptake inhibitors, including cytochrome P-450 enzyme, and serotnin and dopamine transporter and receptor polymorphisms. J Clin Psychopharmacol 2006;26:192–7.

[80] Mihara K, Suzuki A, Kondo T, et al. No relationship between Taq1A polymorphism of dopamine D2 receptor gene and extrapyramidal adverse effects of selective dopamine D2 antagonists, bromperidol, and nemonapride in schizophrenia: a preliminary study (Neuropsych Genetics). Am J Med Genet 2000;96:422–4.

[81] Heils A, Mößner R, Lesch KP. The human serotonin transporter gen polymorphism—basic research and clinical implications. J Neural Transm 1997;104:1005–14.

[82] Caspi A, Sugden K, Moffitt TE, et al. Influence of life stress on depression: moderation by a polymorphism in the 5-HTT gene. Science 2003;301:386–9.

[83] Yu YW, Tsai SJ, Chen TJ, et al. Association study of the serotonin transporter promoter polymorphism and symptomatology and antidepressant response in major depressive disorders. Mol Psychiatry 2002;7(10):1115–9.

[84] Kato M, Ikenaga Y, Wakeno M, et al. Controlled clinical comparison of paroxetine and fluvoxamine considering the serotonin transporter promoter polymorphism. Int Clin Psychopharmacol 2005;20(3):151–6.

[85] Gonda X, Rihmer Z, Juhasz G, et al. High anxiety and migraine are associated with the sallele of the 5HTTLPR gene polymorphism. Psychiatry Res 2007;149(1–3):261–6.

[86] Stein MB, Seedat S, Gelernter J. Serotonin transporter gene promoter polymorphism predicts SSRI response in generalized social anxiety disorder. Psychopharmacol 2006;187:68–72.

[87] Smeraldi E, Zanardi R, Benedetti F, et al. Polymorphism within the promoter of the serotonin transporter gene and antidepresants efficacy of fluvoxamine. Mol Psychiatry 1998;3: 508–11.

[88] Pollock BG, Ferrell RE, Mulsant BH, et al. Allelic variation in the serotonin transporter promoter affects onset of paroxetine treatment response in late-life depression. Neuropsychopharmacology 2000;23(5):587–90.

[89] Zanardi R, Benedetti F, Di Bella D, et al. Efficacy of paroxetine in depression is influenced by a functional polymorphism within the promoter of the serotonin transporter gene. J Clin Psychopharmacol 2000;20:105–7.

[90] Zanardi R, Serretti A, Rossini D, et al. Factors affecting fluvoxamine antidepressant activity: influence of pindolol and 5-HTTLPR in delusional and nondelusional depression. Biol Psychol 2001;50:323–30.

[91] Arias B, Catalan R, Gasto C, et al. 5-HTTLPR polymorphism of the serotonin transporter gene predicts non-remission in major depression patients treated with citalopram in a 12-weeks follow up study. J Clin Psychopharmacol 2003;23:563–7.

[92] Joyce PR, Mulder RT, Luty SE, et al. Age-dependent antidepressant pharmacogenomics: polymorphisms of the serotonin transporter and G protein β3 subunit as predictors of response to fluoxetine and nortryptyline. Int J Neuropsychopharmacol 2003;6:339–46.

[93] Murphy GM Jr, Hollander SB, Rodrigues HE, et al. Effects of the serotonin transporter gene promoter polymorphism on mirtazapine and paroxetine efficacy and adverse events in geriatric major depression. Arch Gen Psychiatry 2004;61:1163–9.

[94] Rausch JL, Johnson ME, Fei YJ, et al. Initial conditions of serotonin transporter kinetics and genotype: influence on SSRI treatment trial outcome. Biol Psychiatry 2002;51:723–32.

[95] Durham LK, Webb SM, Milos PM, et al. The serotonin transporter polymorphism, 5-HTTLPR, is associated with a faster response time to sertraline in an elderly population with major depressive disorder. Psychopharmacology (Berl) 2004;174:525–9.

[96] Hong CJ, Chen TJ, Yu YW, et al. Response to fluoxetine and serotonin 1A receptor (C1019G) polymorphism in Taiwan Chinese major depressive disorder. Pharmacogenomics J 2006;6(1):27–33.

[97] Kim DK, Lim SW, Lee S, et al. Serotonin transporter gene polymorphism and antidepressants response. Neuroreport 2000;11:215–9.

[98] Kim H, Lim SW, Kim S, et al. Monoamine transporter gene polymorphisms and antidepressant response in Koreans with late-life depression. JAMA 2006;296:1609–18.

[99] Yoshida K, Ito K, Sato K, et al. Influence of the serotonin transporter gene-linked polymorphic region on the antidepressants response to fluvoxamine in Japanese depressed patients. Prog Neruopsychopharmacol Biol Psychiatry 2002;26:383–6.

[100] Seretti A, Kato M, De Ronchi D, et al. Meta-analysis of serotonin transporter gene promoter polymorphism (5-HTTLPR) association with selective serotonin reuptake inhibitor efficacy in depressed patients. Mol Psychiatry 2007;12:247–57.

[101] Mundo E, Walker M, Cate T, et al. The role of serotonin transporter protein gene in antidepressant-induced mania in bipolar disorder: preliminary findings. Arch Gen Psychiatry 2001;58:539–44.

[102] Masoliver E, Menoyo A, Perez V, et al. Serotonin transporter linked promoter (polymorphism) in the serotonin transporter gene may be associated with antidepressant-induced mania in bipolar disorder. Psychiatr Genet 2006;16:25–9.

[103] Erdmann J, Shimron-Abarbanell D, Rietschel M. Systematic screening for mutations in the human serotonin-2A 5-HT2A receptor gene: identification of two naturally occurring receptor variants and association analysis in schizophrenia. Hum Genet 1996;97:614–9.

[104] Arranz MJ, Munro J, Own MJ, et al. Evidence for association between polymorphisms in the promoter and coding regions of the 5-HT2A receptor gene and response to clozapine. Mol Psychiatry 1998;3:61–6.

[105] Spurlock G, Helis A, Homas P, et al. A family based association study of T102C polymorphism in 5HT2A and schizophrenia plus identification of new polymorphisms in the promoter. Mol Psychiatry 1998;3:42–9.

[106] McMahon FJ, Buervenich S, Charney D, et al. Variation in the gene encoding the serotonin 2A receptor is associated with outcome of antidepressant treatment. Am J Hum Genet 2006;78(5):804–14.

[107] Cichon S, Nöthen MM, Rietschel M, et al. Pharmacogenetics of schizophrenia. Am J Med Genet 2000;97(1):98–106.

[108] Masellis M, Basile VS, Ozdemir V, et al. Pharmacogenetics of antipsychotic treatment: lessons learned from clozapine. Biol Psychiatry 2000;47(3):252–66.

[109] Chou WH, Yan FX, de Leon J, et al. Extension of a pilot study: impact from the cytochrome P450 2D6 polymorphism on outcome and costs associated with severe mental illness. J Clin Psychopharmacol 2000;20(2):246–51.

ELSEVIER
SAUNDERS

CLINICS IN
LABORATORY
MEDICINE

Clin Lab Med 28 (2008) 645–665

Pharmacogenetic Tests in Asthma Therapy

I-Wen Yu, MS[a],
Bonny Lewis Bukaveckas, PhD[a,b,c,*]

[a]Department of Pharmacy, School of Pharmacy, Virginia Commonwealth University, 410N, 12th Street, P.O. Box 980533, Richmond, VA 23298-0533, USA
[b]Department of Pathology, School of Medicine, Virginia Commonwealth University, PO Box 980662, 1101 E. Marshall Street, Richmond, VA 23298-0662, USA
[c]Department of Anesthesiology, School of Medicine Virginia Commonwealth University, 1200 E. Broad Street, West Hospital, 7th Floor, Rm 7105, Richmond, VA 23219, USA

Background on asthma

Asthma is a common disease worldwide, affecting more than 300 million individuals in the developed world [1]. The incidence of asthma varies in children worldwide from 2.1% in developing countries such as Albania to 32.2% in the United Kingdom (Fig. 1) [2]. In the United States, a trend of increasing asthma prevalence has occurred since 1980, with a possible plateau after 1997, regardless of gender, age, or ethnic group (Fig. 2) [3]. Approximately 7.1% of the United States population—more than 21 million Americans—currently experience asthma.

The United States incidence varies ethnically from 7.3% in white non-Hispanic, 9.4% in black non-Hispanic, to 14.1% in Puerto Ricans [4]. In addition, non-Hispanic blacks are five times more likely to visit the emergency room for asthma exacerbation and three times more likely to be hospitalized and die from asthma than whites. The ethnic differences in prevalence and severity of asthma in the United States could be caused by preexisting risk factors, including genetics, environmental allergen exposure, and socioeconomic level [4].

The high prevalence of asthma comes with a high cost, including 13.9 million outpatient visits, 1.9 million emergency visits, 484,000 hospitalizations, and 4261 deaths from asthma in the United States in 2002 [3]. According to

* Corresponding author. Department of Pharmacy, Virginia Commonwealth University, 410N, 12th Street, P.O. Box 980533, Richmond, VA 23298-0533.
E-mail address: blbukaveckas@vcu.edu (B.L. Bukaveckas).

doi:10.1016/j.cll.2008.05.001   *labmed.theclinics.com*

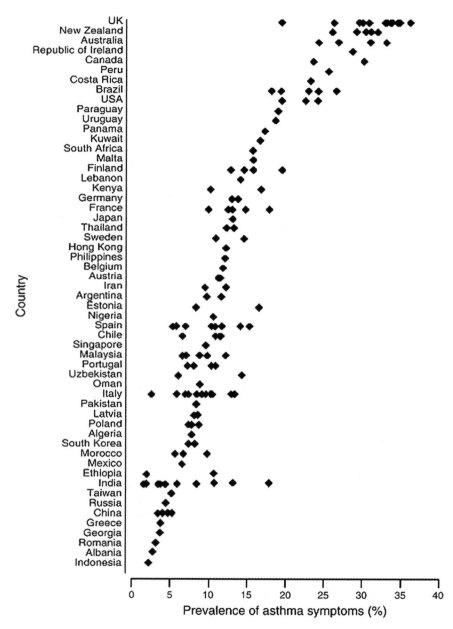

Fig. 1. Worldwide asthma prevalence in children. The prevalence is higher in Western countries than Eastern countries. (*From* Lugogo NL, Kraft M. Epidemiology of asthma. Clin Chest Med 2006;27(1):1–15, v; with permission.)

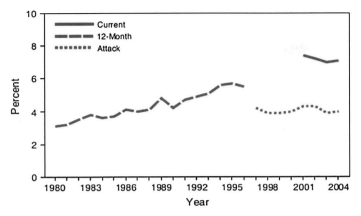

Fig. 2. Prevalence of asthma in United States since 1980. Estimated prevalence of asthma by persons who reported an asthma attack during the preceding 12 months (...), persons who reported having asthma during the preceding 12 months (—), and persons who reported current asthma (—). (*Data from* Moorman JE, Rudd RA, Johnson CA, et al. National Surveillance for Asthma—United States, 1980–2004 [CDC Web site]. Available at: http://www.cdc.gov/mmwr/preview/mmwrhtml/ss5608a1.htm. Accessed March 5, 2008.)

the Asthma and Allergy Foundation, the estimated total annual cost of asthma is more than $18 billion, of which more than half was for medications and health care services [5].

Asthma is a mostly reversible, chronic airway inflammatory disease associated with airflow obstruction, bronchial hyperresponsiveness (BHR), and airway inflammation. Clinical symptoms are cough, wheezing, shortness of breath, and chest tightness caused by mostly reversible airflow obstruction. Inflammation is a key component of asthma.

The pathophysiology of this disease is early-phase inflammation after allergen exposure (Fig. 3), in which increased binding of IgE on mast cells leads to release of mediators, such as histamine, leukotriene, and cytokines, resulting in acute bronchoconstriction. The cytokines from mast cells are likely to recruit more cells to the airway, such as T lymphocytes, eosinophils, neutrophils, and epithelial cells seen in the late phase of inflammation, leading to airway remodeling and incomplete reversibility.

Activation of a specific T-helper cell type 2 (TH2) generates TH2 cytokines interleukin (IL)-4, IL-5, and IL-13, which directly and indirectly target smooth muscle cells and epithelial cells to enhance BHR. In addition, eosinophils that migrate from the circulation into the airway have prolonged survival through IL-5, perpetuating the inflammation and eliciting airway injury. Moreover, repeated cycles of inflammation are followed by ongoing repair processes producing possibly irreversible airway remodeling with hypertrophy of smooth muscle cells, goblet hyperplasia (airway epithelium occupied by goblet cells), and airway wall thickening.

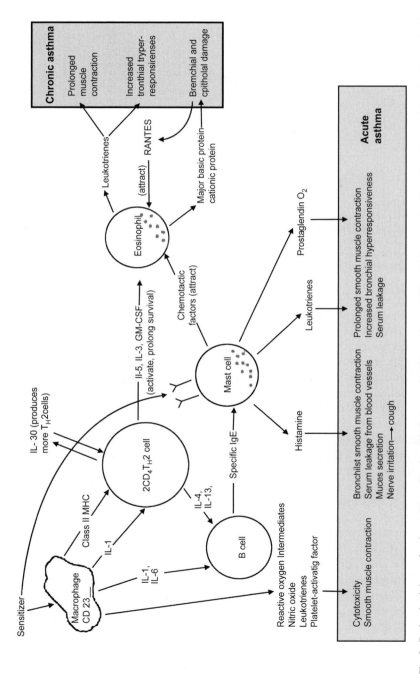

Fig. 3. Pathophysiology of asthma. (*From* Pandya RJ, Solomon G, Kinner A, et al. Diesel exhaust and asthma: hypotheses and molecular mechanisms of action. Environ Health Perspect. 2002;110(Suppl 1):103–12; with permission.)

The degree of inflammation in asthma may vary among individuals because of interaction of genetic and environmental factors [6]. Accordingly, asthma severity is classified as mild, moderate, or severe based on symptoms, lung function, frequency of exacerbation, and physical activity (Table 1).

Pharmacotherapy

Quick-relief drugs, including short-acting β_2-agonists (SABAs) and anticholinergics, treat acute asthma attacks, whereas controllers, including long-acting β_2-agonists (LABAs), inhaled corticosteroids (ICSs), and the leukotriene modifiers, minimize airway inflammation over the long term. The current recommendation for asthma treatment is a stepwise approach based on asthma severity (see Table 1) [7,8].

In step one, pharmacotherapy for mild, intermittent asthma involves a quick-relief drug only for acute symptom control. All other steps also recommend quick-relief drugs in addition to further therapy. Step two includes an additional controller, such as a low-dose ICS, for mild persistent asthma therapy. In step three, either increasing ICS dose or adding one more controller medication, such as an LABA, to the low-to-medium–dose ICS is recommended for moderate persistent asthma. Finally, in step four, high-dose ICS and a LABA are recommended for treating severe persistent asthma. Asthma control should be monitored every 6 months to decide whether to step-up or step-down the pharmacotherapy based on level of symptom control.

Inhaled β_2-agonists are bronchodilators that produce airway smooth muscle relaxation when bound to β_2-adrenergic receptors (β_2ARs). After binding, a cascade of stimulatory G-protein (G_s)–coupled adenyl cyclase activation follows [6]. Based on how rapid the onset and how long the pharmacologic effect lasts, β_2-agonists are characterized either as short-acting (SABA), such as albuterol, metaproterenol, pirbuterol, and levalbuterol, or long-acting (LABA), such as formoterol and salmeterol. In addition to bronchodilation, β_2-agonists protect the airway against hypersensitivity stimuli from exercise, and histamine. The β_2-agonist medications available in the United States as of March 2008 are listed in Table 2.

Pharmacokinetics

SABAs, such as albuterol, are hydrophilic and have onset of action within 5 to 15 minutes after aerosol inhalation, reach peak response within 0.5 to 2 hours, and have a response that is sustained for 4 to 6 hours. Men have a greater volume of distribution for albuterol than women, but African Americans and European Americans have no difference in albuterol pharmacokinetics [9]. In comparison, the onset of bronchodilation is 30 to 50 minutes for LABAs such as salmeterol because of their lipophilicity, a property resulting from the addition of a long side chain. Peak response

Table 1
Stepwise approach for asthma pharmacotherapy

	Mild intermittent	Mild persistent	Moderate persistent	Severe persistent
Symptoms	Symptoms <2 times a week Asymptomatic and normal PEF between exacerbations Exacerbations brief (from a few hours to a few days); intensity may vary	Symptoms >2 times a week but <1 time a day Exacerbations may affect activity	Daily symptoms Daily use of inhaled short-acting β_2-agonist Exacerbations affect activity Exacerbations > 2 times a week; may last days	Continual symptoms Limited physical activity Frequent exacerbations
Nighttime symptoms	<2 times a month	>2 times a month	>1 time a week	Frequent
Lung function	FEV_1 or PEF >80% predicted PEF variability <20%	FEV_1 or PEF >80% predicted PEF variability 20%–30%	FEV_1 or PEF >60%–<80% predicted PEF variability >30%	FEV_1 or PEF <60% predicted PEF variability >30%
Quick Relief	Inhaled short-acting β_2-agonists as needed for symptoms	Inhaled short-acting β_2-agonists as needed for symptoms	Inhaled short-acting β_2-agonists as needed for symptoms	Inhaled short-acting β_2-agonists as needed for symptoms
Long-term control	No daily medication needed	Anti-inflammatory (low-dose ICS), or sustained-release theophylline, or zafirlukast	Anti-inflammatory (medium-dose ICS), or low to medium-dose ICS plus a long-acting bronchodilator or sustained-release theophylline	Anti-inflammatory (high-dose ICS) plus a long-acting bronchodilator or sustained-release theophylline

Four steps, from least to most severe, require increasing medical management. The guidelines recommend that patients are monitored, and if necessary stepped up or down depending on disease control. Current guidelines do not include information on the use of pharmacogenetics in asthma treatment. *Data from* National Asthma Education and Prevention Program Expert Panel. Expert panel report 2: guidelines for the diagnosis and management of asthma. National Institute of Health Publication, Publication Number 97-4051, Bethesda, MD, 1997. Available at: http://www.nhlbi.nih.gov/guidelines/asthma/asthgdln.pdf. Accessed on March 5, 2008; and British Thoracic Society; Scottish Intercollegiate Guidelines Network. British guideline on the management of asthma. Thorax 2003;58(Suppl 1):i1–94.

Table 2
List of β_2-agonist medications available in United States as of March 2008

β_2-agonist (generic)	Brand name
Albuterol	AccuNeb
	ProAir HFA
	Proventil HFA
	Proventil
	Ventolin HFA
	VoSpire ER
Metaproterenol	Alupent
Pirbuterol	Maxair Autohaler
Levalbuterol	Xopenex HFA
	Xopenex
Arformoterol	Brovana
Salmeterol	Serevent Diskus
Fluticasone and salmeterol	Advair Diskus
	Advair HFA
Formoterol	Foradil Aerolizer
Budesonide and formoterol	Symbicort

to LABAs occurs in 2 to 3 hours [10]. The bronchodilatory action of salmeterol lasts for 12 hours. Salmeterol is highly protein-bound and extensively metabolized in the liver. Adverse systemic effects of LABAs are predicted by pharmacokinetics in a dose-dependent relationship [11].

Clinical use

The National Asthma Education and Prevention Program recommends inhaled SABAs be used as needed for acute asthma exacerbation. The usual dose is 360 to 720 μg per four to eight puffs every 20 minutes up to 4 hours for albuterol metered-dose inhaler (MDI). This recommendation contrasts with previous ones for regular use of 180 μg per two puffs for albuterol MDI three to four times daily. Regular use of SABAs has been "a standard approach without the scientific basis since 1970s" [12]. Current guidelines indicate that inhaled LABAs (usual dose, 84 μg per two puffs for salmeterol MDI twice daily) should be combined with ICSs for asthma control, rather than used as a stand-alone therapy.

Measures of response to asthma therapy

In clinical practice, pulmonary function testing is the primary measurement used to assess disease and monitor asthma pharmacotherapy. Pulmonary function testing methods vary. The two most common measures of lung function include forced expiratory volume exhaled in one second (FEV_1) and peak expiratory flow rate (PEF). FEV_1, measured in milliliters, represents the amount of air that patients can forcibly blow out in 1 second.

Response to β_2-agonists can be expressed as the change in FEV_1 from baseline after either a single dose or 12 weeks of treatment. The American Thoracic Society defines an increase of more than 12% and at least 200 mL in FEV_1 as a significant bronchodilator response [7]. An increase of 8% or less is considered within measurement variability. A 12% to 15% increase in FEV_1 is the common arbitrary threshold used in clinical research reports to separate patients who respond well to β_2-agonists from those who respond poorly [13].

Patients can easily measure PEF at home using an inexpensive peak flow meter. PEF is the maximum speed of the air moving out of lung at the beginning of expiration, indicating ventilatory capacity. Because of daily fluctuation, measuring PEF at least twice daily is recommended, preferably on waking and between 5 and 7 hours later to obtain morning and afternoon PEF, respectively. A predicted PEF value of more than 80%, calculated using the Hankinson equation [14] ($b_0 + b_1 \times age + b_2 \times age^2 + b_3 \times height^2$, where the b_0, b_1, b_2, b_3 coefficients vary with age, sex, and race), represents good control of asthma with therapy [7], whereas a value less than 50% indicates the need for short-acting β_2-agonists [7]. In clinical trials, the change of either morning or afternoon PEF from baseline is an end point used to evaluate for treatment effect, although no standard criteria exist for doing so. In one study, a decrease of more than 20% was found to be associated with clinical deterioration of asthma [15].

BHR and exhaled nitric oxide objectively measure the level of airway inflammation. BHR is excessive airway constriction triggered by stimulus. Clinically, a methacholine challenge determines degree of BHR through measuring the doubling concentration of methacholine to cause a 20% decline in FEV_1 (PC_{20}). Therefore, the extent to which asthma pharmacotherapy reduces BHR is occasionally used as a measure of response to anti-inflammatory effect of asthma pharmacotherapy in clinical research. Patients who have more than a three times doubling dose of PC_{20} have been classified good steroid responders [16].

Exhaled nitric oxide was used as the marker of airway inflammation after patients who had asthma were found to have increased levels of exhaled nitric oxide and nitric oxide synthase expression [17]. Exhaled nitric oxide correlated with a "response to steroid," defined as change in pulmonary function testing, asthma symptoms, and BHR [18]. Patients who have symptoms of asthma who respond to steroids have higher exhaled nitric oxide than those who do not, implying inadequate anti-inflammatory treatment. The cutoff of exhaled nitric oxide for steroid response was determined to be approximately 48 parts per billion in one study [18], but no standards are widely used.

For clinical research purposes, subjective measures are used to evaluate the response to β_2-agonists, including rescue use of these agents, symptom score, and asthma quality of life or health outcomes, such as rates of asthma-related emergency visit, hospitalization, and death. These subjective measures are difficult to correlate with the more objective indicators detailed previously because of a lack of correlation studies [19]. Currently, no single absolute indicator exists of response to β_2-agonists for asthma control. A composite score, which considers all ends at once to evaluate response, may be considered [20].

β_2-Agonists are controversial

Concerns remain about the effect of chronic dosing of SABAs or LABAs on mortality and morbidity, specifically occurring in some patients who have unidentified risk factors [21]. From the mid-1960s to early 1980s, several series reported asthma deaths, which were later found to be related to the use of either nonselective β-agonist or high-dose fenoterol in the United Kingdom and New Zealand [22]. The subsequent case-control studies found an increased risk with not only fenoterol but also other β_2-agonists, such as albuterol. Investigators found a higher mortality odds ratio, indicating that these compounds have an association with death and severe exacerbation in asthma [23]. Asthma-related death has been related to excessive use of β-agonists [24].

A link between β_2-agonists and asthma deterioration has been postulated from examination of lung function, BHR, acute exacerbation, and bronchodilator response with treatment. Studies find decreased lung function in patients taking SABAs regularly, whereas lung function is increased in those treated with either SABAs only as needed or regular LABAs [25,26]. PC_{20} equivalent to PD_{20}, indicating the degree of BHR, decreased similarly, possibly indicating a potential for acute exacerbation [25]. Among these studies, some patients taking β_2-agonists experienced poor responses regularly.

Asthma-related death and life-threatening exacerbations occurred in the Salmeterol Multicenter Asthma Research Trial and may have been associated with regular use of salmeterol [27]. These event are rare, but were observed primarily in African Americans. The US Food and Drug Administration has added a black box warning to LABA labels reflecting the observations from this trial. A meta-analysis of 19 clinical trials to evaluate the safety of LABAs concluded that they were associated with increased hospitalization for asthma exacerbation, severe asthma exacerbation, and asthma-related death [28].

Whether adverse outcomes are caused by the detrimental effects of β_2-agonists in a specific group or by disease deterioration from poor response to these agents is still unclear. Estimates show that 60% of the variability between poor and good responders is attributable to genetic causes [29], with a contemporary focus on the β_2-adrenergic receptor gene (ADRB2). Taken together, poor response and adverse outcomes of LABAs and SABAs show a potential factor underlying these responses. Research in β_2-agonist pharmacogenetics is emerging, with a focus on the effect of ADRB2 variants on response or adverse outcomes of β_2-agonists.

β_2-Adrenergic receptor pharmacogenetics

β_2AR, the target of β_2-agonists, is a G protein-coupled receptor with seven transmembrane segments and 413 amino acids. As shown in Fig. 4, this receptor has three extracellular and three intracellular loops. The active sites in β_2AR for β_2-agonist binding include aspartate residue 113, serine residues 204 and 207, and asparagine residue 293 [30]. Activation of β_2AR with β_2-agonist binding uncouples stimulatory G proteins, followed by activation of adenyl cyclase, which converts ATP to cyclic AMP (cAMP) and activates protein kinase A (Fig. 5). Increased cAMP levels and phosphorylated proteins by protein kinase A indirectly cause relaxation of bronchial smooth muscle and mast cell stabilization. Desensitization of this pathway begins with the uncoupling of β_2AR from adenylate cyclase as an

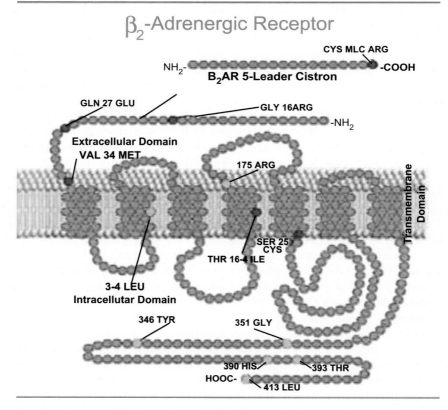

Fig. 4. β_2AR with seven transmembrane domains. Nonsynonymous coding variants are shown in red and synonymous variants are shown in yellow. (*From* Liggett SB. Polymorphisms of the beta2-adrenergic receptor and asthma. Am J Respir Crit Care Med. 1997;156:S156–62.)

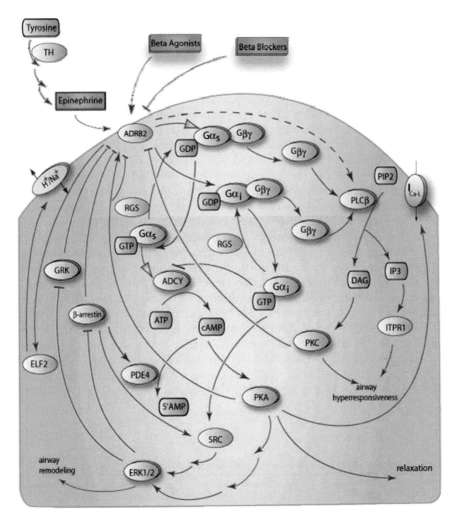

Fig. 5. The physiologic and pharmacologic pathway of β_2 agonist on β_2AR. This pathway is complex and many signal cascade proteins shown may have relevant genetic variations that may modify sensitivity to pharmacotherapy. (*From* Johnson M. Molecular mechanisms of beta(2)-adrenergic receptor function, response, and regulation. J Allergy Clin Immunol 2006;117:18–24; with permission.)

autoregulation process in response to excessive exposure to β_2-agonists [31]. Prolonged exposure to β_2-agonists results in internalization of β_2AR, causing decreased receptor number on the cell surface. Within this pharmacologic pathway, the genes that encode the proteins involved in this process could be considered candidate genes affecting the response to β_2-agonists.

ADRB2 was first cloned by Kobilka and colleagues [32]. The intronless gene contains 2011 nucleotide base pairs on the long arm of chromosome 5 (5q31–32). *ADRB2*, encoding β_2AR, is transcribed from the forward strand. A total of 49 single nucleotide polymorphisms (SNPs) have been identified in the region, spanning from 3470 bp upstream to 1866 bp after the stop codon [33]. The 10 polymorphisms [34,35] listed in Table 3 are functional SNPs, defined as a change in amino acid or expression of β_2AR. Coding SNPs at nucleotides 46, 79, and 491 (46A → G, 79C → G, and 491T → C) result in arginine substitution for glycine (Arg16 → Gly) and glutamine substitution for glutamic acid (Gln27 → Glu) of the *N*-terminus and threonine substitution for isoleucine (Thr164 → Ile) of transmembrane domain [36]. A noncoding SNP within the 5′ promoter, −47T → C, in amino acid residual 19 of the 19-amino acid β upstream peptide affects β_2AR expression [37]. Two other nonsynonymous SNPs (−468C → G and −654G → A) in the upstream region may affect transcription of β_2AR [38]. The frequency of *ADRB2* alleles varies with ethnicity, as summarized in Tables 4 and 5. A higher proportion of Asians and Africans have alternative alleles for the Arg19 → Gys, Arg16 → Gly, and Gln27 → Glu polymorphisms compared with European Americans [39]. The Ile164 allele is only and rarely (<1%) observed in European Americans, and 15% to 27% of Caucasians and 24% of African Americans are homozygous Arg16 (see Table 5) [40]. In addition, for people of African decent, the linkage disequilibrium analysis shows three SNP blocks, including functional SNPs. The first block is from −654 to −468 and shows strong linkage disequilibrium; the second block is from −20 to −47, again showing strong linkage

Table 3
List of functional single nucleotide polymorphisms on *ADRB2*

dbSNP rs No.	Nucleotide No.	Variant/reference allele	Function	Amino acid No.	Variant/reference amino acid
rs12654778	−654	A/G	Transcription of ADRB2		
rs11168070	−468	G/C	Transcription of ADRB2		
rs1042711	−47	T/C	BUP		Cys [C]/Arg [R]
rs33973603		G/A		15	Ser [S]/Asn [N]
rs1042713	46	A/G	β_2AR	16	Arg [R]/Gly [G]
rs1042714	79	C/G	β_2AR	27	Gln [Q]/Glu [E]
rs1800888	491	T/C	β_2AR	164	Ile [I]/Thr [T]
rs3729943	659	G/C	β_2AR	220	Cys [C]/Ser [S]
rs41320345		C/T	β_2AR	240	Leu [L]/Phe [F]
rs41358746		T/G	β_2AR	247	His [H]/Gln [Q]

This list was assembled using NCBI Entrez SNP, dbSNP BUILD 128. *Abbreviations:* dbSNP rs No, single nucleotide polymorphism database reference cluster number; ADRB2, beta-2-adrenergic receptor, surface.

Table 4
Frequency of alleles and genotypes in ADRB2 from HapMap data

%	rs12654778 (−654G/A)					rs11168070 (−468G/C)					rs1042711 (−47C/T)				
	G	A	GG	AG	AA	G	C	GG	CG	CC	C	T	CC	CT	TT
CEU	66.4	33.6	44.8	43.1	12.1	na	na	na	na	na	na	na	na	na	na
CHB	64.4	35.6	37.8	53.3	8.9	12.2	87.8	0	24.4	75.6	4.9	95.1	0	9.8	90.2
JPT	66.7	33.3	48.7	35.9	15.4	8	92	2.3	11.4	86.4	6	94	2.4	7.1	90.5
YRI	79.7	20.3	66.1	27.1	6.8	16.9	83.1	5.1	23.7	71.2	12.3	87.7	1.9	20.8	77.4

%	rs1042713 (46G/A)					rs1042714 (79G/C)					rs1800888 (491C/T)				
	G	A	GG	AG	AA	G	C	GG	CG	CC	C	T	CC	CT	TT
CEU	67.5	32.5	46.7	41.7	11.7	46.7	53.3	31.7	30	38.3	99.2	0.8	98.3	1.7	0
CHB	46.7	53.3	20	53.3	26.7	12.2	87.8	0	24.4	75.6	100	0	100	0	0
JPT	61.4	38.6	36.4	50	13.6	8	92	2.3	11.4	86.4	100	0	100	0	0
YRI	52.5	47.5	33.3	38.3	28.3	17.5	82.5	5	25	70	100	0	100	0	0

%	rs3729943														
	C	G	CC	CG	GG										
CEU	100	0	100	0	0	—	—	—	—	—	—	—	—	—	—
CHB	100	0	100	0	0	—	—	—	—	—	—	—	—	—	—
JPT	100	0	100	0	0	—	—	—	—	—	—	—	—	—	—
YRI	94.8	5.2	89.7	10.3	0	—	—	—	—	—	—	—	—	—	—

Of note is the ethnic variation in minor allele frequency of rs1042713 (in bold), which codes for the Gly16→Arg polymorphism. This polymorphism has been linked with variable response to chronic therapy with β2 agonist medications. CEU, CEPH (Utah residents with ancestry from northern and western Europe); CHB, Han Chinese in Beijing, China; YRI, Yoruba in Ibadan, Nigeria; JPT, Japanese in Tokyo, Japan.

Table 5

Frequency of allele and genotype of single nucleotide polymorphism rs1042713, coding for the Arg16→Gly polymorphism on ADRB2 among different ethnic populations

| Population | n^a | Genotype frequency | | | Allele frequency | |
		Arg^b	Arg/Gly	Gly^c	Arg16 (95% CI)	Gly16 (95% CI)
Ghanaian	100	0.27	0.53	0.20	0.54 (0.46–0.60)	0.46 (0.39–0.54)
Kenyan	100	0.35	0.44	0.21	0.57 (0.50–0.64)	0.43 (0.36–0.50)
Sudanese	52	0.12	0.63	0.25	0.43 (0.34–0.53)	0.57 (0.47–0.66)
Filipino	78	0.29	0.50	0.20	0.54 (0.46–0.62)	0.46 (0.38–0.54)
Chinese	99	0.33	0.51	0.16	0.58 (0.51–0.65)	0.42 (0.35–0.49)
Chinese (18)	104	0.36	0.46	0.18	0.59 (0.49–0.68)	0.41 (0.32–0.51)
African American (18)	123	0.24	0.50	0.26	0.49 (0.40–0.58)	0.51 (0.42–0.60)
Saudi	100	0.18	0.58	0.24	0.47 (0.40–0.54)	0.53 (0.46–0.60)
Indian (Southwest Asia)	99	0.36	0.36	0.28	0.55 (0.47–0.62)	0.45 (0.38–0.53)
Scottish (Europe)	100	0.23	0.36	0.41	0.41 (0.34–0.48)	0.59 (0.52–0.66)
Caucasian United States (15)	212	0.15	0.46	0.39	0.38 (0.34–0.45)	0.62 (0.55–0.68)
Caucasian United States (18)	188	0.27	0.38	0.35	0.46 (0.39–0.53)	0.54 (0.47–0.61)
Swedish (Europe) (52)	180	0.19	0.44	0.37	0.41 (0.55–0.69)	0.59 (0.52–0.66)

[a] Number of subjects.
[b] Homozygous.
[c] Homozygous Gly16.

(*Data from* Maxwell TJ, Ameyaw MM, Pritchard S, et al. Beta-2 beta(2)-adrenergic receptor genotypes and haplotypes in different ethnic groups. Int J Mol Med 2005;16:573–80.)

disequilibrium; and the third block includes 46 and 79 in strong linkage disequilibrium. In the population of European decent, one haplotype block stretches from −654 to 79. Experts have observed that 48% of Caucasians have haplotype Arg19Gly16Glu27Thr164, whereas 55% of African Americans have Cys19Arg16Gln27Thr164.

In vitro studies using transfected cell lines with expressed β_2AR showed that the Gly16 receptor had an enhanced agonist-promoted down-regulation relative to Arg16 [41]; a greater concentration of β_2-agonist was needed to down-regulate Glu27 receptor compared with Gln27 [42]. As shown in Fig. 6, the Gly16Gln27 receptors had the lowest expression, indicating the highest extent of postagonist down-regulation, whereas Arg16Glu27 receptors, which have not been observed in vivo, had the highest extent of expression, indicating resistance to down-regulation in vitro [41].

The upstream promoter region of *ADRB2* has received less attention. Only the Arg19→Cys polymorphism has been studied in vitro. β_2AR density, as quantified by [^{125}I] CYP radioligand binding, was greater within Cys19 than Arg19 in COS-7 cell model and primary culture of human airway smooth muscle cells [49].

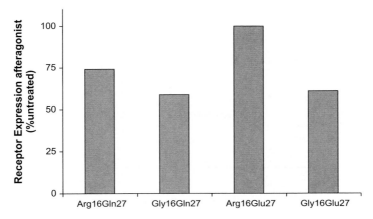

Fig. 6. In vitro β_2AR expression. Relative expression of on β_2AR in transgenic cells after exposure to β-agonist varies according to genotype at positions 16 and 27. Expression is relative to untreated cells of the same genotype. (*Data from* McGraw DW, Forbes SL, Kramer LA, et al. Polymorphisms of the 5′ leader cistron of the human beta2-beta(2)-adrenergic receptor regulate receptor expression. J Clin Invest 1998;102:1927–32.)

In vivo acute response to β_2-agonists

Martinez and colleagues [13] performed spirometry in 269 children who had a history of wheezing and those who did not, before and after inhaled 180 µg of albuterol. A 15.3% improvement in FEV_1 was used to define a positive response in this study. When compared with homozygous Gly16, Arg16 homozygotes were 5.3 times (95% CI, 1.6–17.7) more likely to respond acutely to albuterol. When compared with homozygous Glu27, homozygotes for Gln27 were 3.1 times (95% CI, 0.8–11.4) more likely to respond to albuterol, but the association was not significant. Similarly, Arg16 carrier status was associated with a greater bronchodilator response in Puerto Ricans [43]. An in vivo finding that Arg16 carriers have a greater acute bronchodilator response in some populations is consistent with contradicts the in vitro finding that Gly16 receptor is prone to down-regulation after agonist exposure, but not the case in Asian Indians.

In 80 Asian Indians who had stable asthma, Kukreti and colleagues [44] found that patients who had the homozygous Arg16 genotype were good responders with a probability of 7.3% ($x = 3$), whereas poor responders had a probability of 33.3% ($x = 13$), indicating that good bronchodilator responders are unlikely to have the Arg16 allele. Tsai and colleagues [45] reported a significant association between Arg19→Cys polymorphism, rather than Arg16→Gly, and bronchodilator drug response among 264 African American children who had asthma. Cys19 carriers had lower bronchodilator response compared with Arg19 carriers.

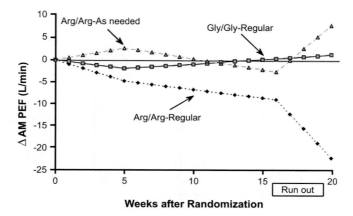

Weeks after Randomization

Fig. 7. Regular β-agonist treatment caused decreased lung function in β_2AR 16Arg homozygotes. Morning PEF in Arg16 homozygous patients decreased steadily with regular treatment, in contrast to Gly16 homozygous patients who maintained lung function with this regimen. Arg16 homozygotes maintained lung function over time with as-needed β-agonist. (*From* Taylor DR, Drazen JM, Herbison GP, et al. Asthma exacerbations during long term beta agonist use: influence of beta(2) adrenoceptor polymorphism. Thorax 2000;55:762–7; with permission.)

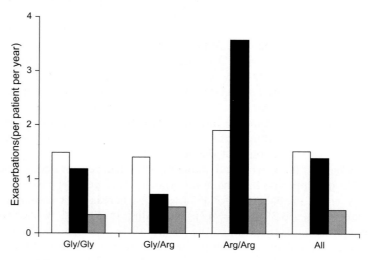

Fig. 8. Asthma exacerbations by *ADRB2* genotype. Total asthma exacerbation in patients who had different genotype and one different β_2-agonist treatment of either placebo (*white*), albuterol (*blue*), or salmeterol (*black*).

Response to chronic dosing with β₂-agonists is genotype-dependant

Israel and colleagues [35] performed retrospective genotyping of 190 subjects who had mild asthma randomized to albuterol as-needed or two puffs
four times a day. These patients were a subset of the population in the Beta
Agonist in Mild Asthma Study. As shown in Fig. 7, Arg16 homozygous
asthmatics on regular albuterol for 16 weeks had reduced morning peak
flows from baseline, whereas homozygous Gly16 asthmatics taking regular
albuterol retained increased morning peak flows. In addition, the morning
peak flows of homozygous Arg16 asthmatics on regular albuterol fell
31 L/min from those of homozygous Arg16 asthmatics on as-needed albuterol. Small and colleagues [46] proposed that because Arg16 receptors
have a lower degree of desensitization due to endogenous agonists, they
have a higher degree of desensitization due to exogenous agonists.

Taylor and colleagues [47] showed that homozygous Arg16 asthmatics
taking 400 µg albuterol Diskhaler four times a day for 24 weeks had a higher
rate of asthma exacerbation than those taking placebo (Fig. 8). Regular

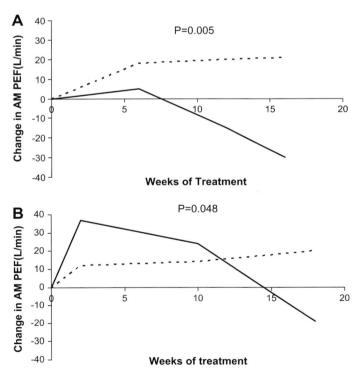

Fig. 9. Change of morning PEF in β₂AR Arg16 homozygous and Gly16 homozygous subjects
who received (*A*) salmeterol compared with placebo along treatment period and (*B*) salmeterol
combined with ICS along treatment period. (*Data from* Wechsler ME, Lehman E, Lazarus SC,
et al. Beta-adrenergic receptor polymorphisms and response to salmeterol. Am J Respir Crit
Care Med 2006;173:519–26.)

albuterol treatment in homozygous Arg16 asthmatics resulted in a higher rate of asthma exacerbation compared with other subjects who were not homozygous for Arg16. However, these differences were not observed with salmeterol.

In summary, β_2AR Arg16 homozygotes may be associated with decreased lung function and increased asthma exacerbation with regular SABA use. Subsequently, to determine the effect of Arg16→Gly polymorphism on response to salmeterol monotherapy, Wechsler and colleagues [48] genotyped 43 patients who had persistent asthma who were receiving salmeterol 42 µg twice daily for 16 weeks. Within 16 weeks of treatment, morning PEF increased in subjects who had the Gly16→Gly polymorphism receiving salmeterol compared with those taking placebo, whereas it decreased in subjects homozygous for Arg16 (Fig. 9A). The difference in morning PEF among genotype groups at the end of treatment reached 51 l per minute.

Furthermore, 30 more patients receiving salmeterol combined with ICS were genotyped. As shown in Fig. 9B, after 2 weeks of treatment, morning PEF deteriorated in Arg16 homozygous individuals but steadily increased in Gly16 homozygotes. Therefore, β_2AR Arg16 may be associated with decreased lung function in the regular use of LABA with or without ICS. Whether this deterioration has clinical implications, meaning an increase of asthma exacerbation or hospitalization, must be confirmed in follow-up studies. Avoiding bronchodilator treatment with regular use of salmeterol may be appropriate for asthmatics who have the Arg16 homozygous genotype.

Summary

The β_2AR genotypes, including the Arg16→Gly polymorphism, may have therapeutic significance for asthmatics undergoing β_2-agonist treatment, although the gap between acute response and chronic effect of β_2-agonists remains unanswered. Pharmacogenetic effects are likely not limited to this one SNP, or even this one gene. Causality between this SNP and outcomes must be evaluated in prospective treatment studies. In addition, Caucasians are the main study population in most association studies for long-term β_2-agonist treatment. Therefore, information on the role of genetic variation on asthma therapeutic outcomes in a more diverse population sample must be collected.

Acknowledgments

The authors wish to acknowledge Drs. Anne-Marie Irani and Lawrence Schwartz for their interest and enthusiasm in the use of genetic testing in the care of asthma patients.

References

[1] "10 Facts on asthma" World Health Organization fact file. Available at: http://www.who. int/features/factfiles/asthma/en/index.html. [Accessed on March 14, 2008].

[2] Lugogo NL, Kraft M. Epidemiology of asthma. Clin Chest Med 2006;27(1):1–15, v.

[3] National Surveillance for Asthma—United States, 1980–2004 CDC report. Available at: http://www.cdc.gov/mmwr/preview/mmwrhtml/ss5608a1.htm. [Accessed on March 5, 2008].

[4] Centers for Disease Control and Prevention. Asthma prevalence and control characteristics by race/ethnicity-United States, 2002. MMWR Morb Mortal Wkly Rep 2004;53:145–8.

[5] Cost of asthma. Available at: http://www.aafa.org/display.cfm?id=6&;sub = 63&cont = 252 [Accessed on March 5, 2008].

[6] Kelly WH, Sorkness CA. Asthma. In: Dipiro JT, Talbert RL, Yee GC, et al, editors. Pharmacotherapy: a pathophysiologic approach. 5th edition. New York: McGraw Hill; 2002. p. 475–510.

[7] National Asthma Education and Prevention Program Expert Panel. Expert panel report 2: guidelines for the diagnosis and management of asthma. National Institute of Health Publication, Publication Number 97-4051, Bethesda, MD, 1997. Available at: http://www. nhlbi.nih.gov/guidelines/asthma/asthgdln.pdf. [Accessed on March 5, 2008]

[8] British Thoracic Society; Scottish Intercollegiate Guidelines Network. British guideline on the management of asthma. Thorax 2003;58(Suppl 1):i1–94.

[9] Mohamed MH, Lima JJ, Eberle LV, et al. Effects of gender and race on albuterol pharmacokinetics. Pharmacotherapy 1999;19:157–61.

[10] Serevent Diskus prescribing information. Available at: http://us.gsk.com/products/assets/ us_serevent_diskus.pdf. [Accessed on March 5, 2008].

[11] Whelna GJ, Szefler SJ. Asthma management. In: Burton ME, Shaw LM, Schentag JJ, Evans WE, editors. Applied pharmacokinetics & pharmacodynamics principles of therapeutic drug monitoring. 4th edition. Baltimore, MD: Lippincott Williams & Wilkins; 2006. p. 259–83.

[12] Taylor DR, Sears MR, Cockcroft DW. The beta-agonist controversy. Med Clin North Am 1996;80:719–48.

[13] Martinez FD, Graves PE, Baldini M, et al. Association between genetic polymorphisms of the beta2-adrenoceptor and response to albuterol in children with and without a history of wheezing. J Clin Invest 1997;100:3184–8.

[14] Hankinson J, Odencrantz J, Fedan KB. Spirometric reference values from a sample of the general US population. Am J Respir Crit Care Med 1999;159(1):179–87.

[15] Chervinsky P, van As A, Bronsky EA, et al. Fluticasone propionate aerosol for the treatment of adults with mild to moderate asthma. The Fluticasone Propionate Asthma Study Group. J Allergy Clin Immunol 1994;94(4):676–83.

[16] Szefler SJ, Martin RJ, King TS, et al. Significant variability in response to inhaled corticosteroids for persistent asthma. J Allergy Clin Immunol 2002;109:410–8.

[17] Kharitonov SA, Yates D, Robbins RA, et al. Increased nitric oxide in exhaled air of asthmatic patients. Lancet 1994;343:133–5.

[18] Smith AD, Cowan JO, Brassett KP, et al. Exhaled nitric oxide: a predictor of steroid response. Am J Respir Crit Care Med 2005;172:453–9.

[19] Zhang J, Yu C, Holgate ST, et al. Variability and lack of predictive ability of asthma endpoints in clinical trials. Eur Respir J 2002;20:1102–9.

[20] Bateman ED, Boushey HA, Bousquet J, et al. Can guideline-defined asthma control be achieved? The gaining optimal asthma control study. Am J Respir Crit Care Med 2004; 170:836–44.

[21] Salpeter SR, Ormiston TM, Salpeter EE. Meta-analysis: respiratory tolerance to regular beta2-agonist use in patients with asthma. Ann Intern Med 2004;140(10):802–13.

[22] Crane J, Pearce N, Flatt A, et al. Prescribed fenoterol and death from asthma in New Zealand, 1981–83: case-control study. Lancet 1989;1:917–22.

[23] Spitzer WO, Suissa S, Ernst P, et al. The use of beta-agonists and the risk of death and near death from asthma. N Engl J Med 1992;326:501–6.

[24] Suissa S, Ernst P, Boivin JF, et al. A cohort analysis of excess mortality in asthma and the use of inhaled beta-agonists. Am J Respir Crit Care Med 1994;149:604–10.

[25] Taylor DR, Sears MR, Herbison GP, et al. Regular inhaled beta agonist in asthma: effects on exacerbations and lung function. Thorax 1993;48:134–8.

[26] van Schayck CP, Cloosterman SG, Bijl-Hofland ID, et al. Is the increase in bronchial responsiveness or FEV1 shortly after cessation of beta2-agonists reflecting a real deterioration of the disease in allergic asthmatic patients? A comparison between short-acting and long-acting beta2-agonists. Respir Med 2002;96:155–62.

[27] Nelson HS, Weiss ST, Bleecker ER, et al. The Salmeterol Multicenter Asthma Research Trial: a comparison of usual pharmacotherapy for asthma or usual pharmacotherapy plus salmeterol. Chest 2006;129:15–26.

[28] Salpeter SR, Buckley NS, Ormiston TM, et al. Meta-analysis: effect of long-acting beta-agonists on severe asthma exacerbations and asthma-related deaths. Ann Intern Med 2006;144:904–12.

[29] Drazen JM, Silverman EK, Lee TH, et al. Heterogeneity of therapeutic responses in asthma. Br Med Bull 2000;56:1054–70.

[30] Kobilka BK, Kobilka TS, Daniel K, et al. Chimeric alpha 2-,beta 2-adrenergic receptors: delineation of domains involved in effector coupling and ligand binding specificity. Science 1988;240(4857):1310–6.

[31] Johnson M. Molecular mechanisms of beta(2)-beta(2)-adrenergic receptor function, response, and regulation. J Allergy Clin Immunol 2006;117:18–24, quiz 25.

[32] Kobilka BK, MacGregor C, Daniel K, et al. Functional activity and regulation of human beta 2-adrenergic receptors expressed in Xenopus oocytes. J Biol Chem 1987;262(32): 15796–802.

[33] Hawkins GA, Tantisira K, Meyers DA, et al. Sequence, haplotype, and association analysis of ADRbeta2 in a multiethnic asthma case-control study. Am J Respir Crit Care Med 2006; 174:1101–9.

[34] NCBI dbSNP SNP linked to Gene ADRB2 (geneID:154) Via Contig Annotation. Available at: http://www.ncbi.nlm.nih.gov/SNP/snp_ref.cgi?locusId=154 [Accessed on March 5, 2008].

[35] Israel E, Drazen JM, Liggett SB, et al. The effect of polymorphisms of the beta(2)-adrenergic receptor on the response to regular use of albuterol in asthma. Am J Respir Crit Care Med 2000;162:75–80.

[36] Reihsaus E, Innis M, MacIntyre N, et al. Mutations in the gene encoding for the beta 2-adrenergic receptor in normal and asthmatic subjects. Am J Respir Cell Mol Biol 1993;8: 334–9.

[37] McGraw DW, Forbes SL, Kramer LA, et al. Polymorphisms of the 5' leader cistron of the human beta2-adrenergic receptor regulate receptor expression. J Clin Invest 1998;102: 1927–32.

[38] Drysdale CM, McGraw DW, Stack CB, et al. Complex promoter and coding region beta 2-adrenergic receptor haplotypes alter receptor expression and predict in vivo responsiveness. Proc Natl Acad Sci U S A 2000;97:10483–8.

[39] HapMap data Rel22. Available at: http://www.hapmap.org/cgi-perl/gbrowse/hapmap_B36/. [Accessed on March 5, 2008].

[40] Maxwell TJ, Ameyaw MM, Pritchard S, et al. Beta-2 adrenergic receptor genotypes and haplotypes in different ethnic groups. Int J Mol Med 2005;16:573–80.

[41] Green SA, Turki J, Innis M, et al. Amino-terminal polymorphisms of the human beta 2-adrenergic receptor impart distinct agonist-promoted regulatory properties. Biochemistry 1994;33:9414–9.

[42] Green SA, Turki J, Bejarano P, et al. Influence of beta 2-adrenergic receptor genotypes on signal transduction in human airway smooth muscle cells. Am J Respir Cell Mol Biol 1995;13:25–33.

[43] Choudhry S, Ung N, Avila PC, et al. Pharmacogenetic differences in response to albuterol between Puerto Ricans and Mexicans with asthma. Am J Respir Crit Care Med 2005;171: 563–70.

[44] Kukreti R, Bhatnagar P, B-Rao C, et al. Beta (2)-adrenergic receptor polymorphisms and response to salbutamol among Indian asthmatics*. Pharmacogenomics 2005;6:399–410.

[45] Tsai HJ, Shaikh N, Kho JY, et al. Beta 2-adrenergic receptor polymorphisms: pharmacogenetic response to bronchodilator among African American asthmatics. Hum Genet 2006; 119:547–57.

[46] Small KM, McGraw DW, Liggett SB. Pharmacology and physiology of human adrenergic receptor polymorphisms. Annu Rev Pharmacol Toxicol 2003;43:381–411.

[47] Taylor DR, Drazen JM, Herbison GP, et al. Asthma exacerbations during long term beta agonist use: influence of beta(2) adrenoceptor polymorphism. Thorax 2000;55:762–7.

[48] Wechsler ME, Lehman E, Lazarus SC, et al. Beta-adrenergic receptor polymorphisms and response to salmeterol. Am J Respir Crit Care Med 2006;173:519–26.

ELSEVIER
SAUNDERS

CLINICS IN
LABORATORY
MEDICINE

Clin Lab Med 28 (2008) 667–672

Index

Note: Page numbers of article titles are in **boldface** type.

A

Addiction, to opioids, 585–588

ADRB2 gene polymorphisms, asthma therapy and, 656–658

Adverse drug reactions, 493
to opioids, 584–585
to schizophrenia therapy, 628–629
to warfarin, 519, 540

Affymetrix GeneChip, 600

Agranulocytosis, clozapine-induced, pharmacogenetic testing for, 601, 607–608

Albuterol, for asthma
acute response to, 659–662
brand names for, 651
controversy over, 653
dose for, 651
pharmacokinetics of, 649

Aldehyde dehydrogenase gene polymorphisms, 505

Alfentanil, pharmacogenetics of, 590

Amitriptyline, pharmacogenetics-guided dose modifications for, 621–623

Amphetamines, pharmacogenetics of, 605

AmpliChip CYP450 Test, 601, 606, 610

Analgesia response, genetic factors in, 573–576

Anticoagulants. *See* Warfarin.

Antidepressants
adverse effects of, 629–631
pharmacogenetics of, 604–605
pharmacogenetics-guided dose modifications for, **619–626**
clinical implications of, 621–622
cytochrome P450 gene polymorphisms and, 621–624
limitations of, 620–621
rationale for, 619–620
with tamoxifen, 561

Arformoterol, for asthma, 651

Aripiprazole, pharmacogenetics of, 604

Aromatase inhibitors, for breast cancer prevention, 562

Asthma, **645–665**
clinical features of, 647
drug therapy for
beta agonists, 649–662
pharmacokinetics of, 649, 651
response to, measures of, 650–652
stepwise approach to, 650
types of, 649
epidemiology of, 645–647
pathophysiology of, 647–649

Atomoxetine, pharmacogenetics of, 605

B

Back pain, genetic factors in, 570–571

Beta-agonists, for asthma, 649–662
controversy over, 653
in stepwise approach, 650
list of, 651
pharmacogenetics of, 654–662
pharmacokinetics of, 649, 651
response to, 651–653, 659–662

BRCA genes, 503, 507–508

Breast cancer
genetic markers of, 503, 507–508
tamoxifen for. *See* Tamoxifen.

Bronchial hyperresponsiveness, for asthma therapy measurement, 652–653

Budesonide, for asthma, 651

Bupropion, pharmacogenetics-guided dose modifications for, 621

Butorphanol, administration routes for, 585

Butyrophenones, for schizophrenia, 628

0272-2712/08/$ - see front matter © 2008 Elsevier Inc. All rights reserved.
doi:10.1016/S0272-2712(08)00065-6
labmed.theclinics.com

United States Postal Service
Statement of Ownership, Management, and Circulation
(All Periodicals Publications Except Requestor Publications)

1. Publication Title
Clinics in Laboratory Medicine

2. Publication Number
0 0 0 - 7 1 3

3. Filing Date
9/15/08

4. Issue Frequency
Mar, Jun, Sep, Dec

5. Number of Issues Published Annually
4

6. Annual Subscription Price
$189.00

7. Complete Mailing Address of Known Office of Publication *(Not printer)* *(Street, city, county, state, and ZIP+4)*
Elsevier Inc.
360 Park Avenue South
New York, NY 10010-1710

Contact Person
Stephen Bushing

Telephone *(Include area code)*
215-239-3688

8. Complete Mailing Address of Headquarters or General Business Office of Publisher *(Not printer)*
Elsevier Inc., 360 Park Avenue South, New York, NY 10010-1710

9. Full Names and Complete Mailing Addresses of Publisher, Editor, and Managing Editor *(Do not leave blank)*
Publisher *(Name and complete mailing address)*
John Schrefer, Elsevier, Inc., 1600 John F. Kennedy Blvd. Suite 1800, Philadelphia, PA 19103-2899

Editor *(Name and complete mailing address)*
Joanne Husovski, Elsevier, Inc., 1600 John F. Kennedy Blvd. Suite 1800, Philadelphia, PA 19103-2899

Managing Editor *(Name and complete mailing address)*
Catherine Bewick, Elsevier, Inc., 1600 John F. Kennedy Blvd. Suite 1800, Philadelphia, PA 19103-2899

10. Owner *(Do not leave blank. If the publication is owned by a corporation, give the name and address of the corporation immediately followed by the names and addresses of all stockholders owning or holding 1 percent or more of the total amount of stock. If not owned by a corporation, give the names and addresses of the individual owners. If owned by a partnership or other unincorporated firm, give its name and address as well as those of each individual owner. If the publication is published by a nonprofit organization, give its name and address.)*

Full Name	Complete Mailing Address
Wholly owned subsidiary of	4520 East-West Highway
Reed/Elsevier, US holdings	Bethesda, MD 20814

11. Known Bondholders, Mortgagees, and Other Security Holders Owning or Holding 1 Percent or More of Total Amount of Bonds, Mortgages, or Other Securities. If none, check box ☐ None

Full Name	Complete Mailing Address
N/A	

12. Tax Status *(For completion by nonprofit organizations authorized to mail at nonprofit rates)* *(Check one)*
The purpose, function, and nonprofit status of this organization and the exempt status for federal income tax purposes:
☐ Has Not Changed During Preceding 12 Months
☐ Has Changed During Preceding 12 Months *(Publisher must submit explanation of change with this statement)*

PS Form 3526, September 2006 (Page 1 of 3) (Instructions Page 3)) PSN 7530-01-000-9931 **PRIVACY NOTICE:** See our Privacy policy in www.usps.com

13. Publication Title
Clinics in Laboratory Medicine

14. Issue Date for Circulation Data Below
June 2008

15. Extent and Nature of Circulation

		Average No. Copies Each Issue During Preceding 12 Months	No. Copies of Single Issue Published Nearest to Filing Date
a. Total Number of Copies *(Net press run)*		1250	1100
b. Paid Circulation (By Mail and Outside the Mail)	(1) Mailed Outside-County Paid Subscriptions Stated on PS Form 3541. *(Include paid distribution above nominal rate, advertiser's proof copies, and exchange copies)*	444	402
	(2) Mailed In-County Paid Subscriptions Stated on PS Form 3541 *(Include paid distribution above nominal rate, advertiser's proof copies, and exchange copies)*		
	(3) Paid Distribution Outside the Mails Including Sales Through Dealers and Carriers, Street Vendors, Counter Sales, and Other Paid Distribution Outside USPS®	193	182
	(4) Paid Distribution by Other Classes Mailed Through the USPS *(e.g. First-Class Mail®)*		
c. Total Paid Distribution *(Sum of 15b (1), (2), (3), and (4))* ▶		637	584
d. Free or Nominal Rate Distribution (By Mail and Outside the Mail)	(1) Free or Nominal Rate Outside-County Copies Included on PS Form 3541	67	50
	(2) Free or Nominal Rate In-County Copies Included on PS Form 3541		
	(3) Free or Nominal Rate Copies Mailed at Other Classes Mailed Through the USPS (e.g. First-Class Mail)		
	(4) Free or Nominal Rate Distribution Outside the Mail (Carriers or other means)		
e. Total Free or Nominal Rate Distribution *(Sum of 15d (1), (2), (3) and (4))* ▶		67	50
f. Total Distribution *(Sum of 15c and 15e)* ▶		704	634
g. Copies not Distributed *(See instructions to publishers #4 (page #3))* ▶		546	466
h. Total *(Sum of 15f and g)* ▶		1250	1100
i. Percent Paid (15c divided by 15f times 100) ▶		90.48%	92.11%

16. Publication of Statement of Ownership
☐ If the publication is a general publication, publication of this statement is required. Will be printed in the **December 2008** issue of this publication.
☐ Publication not required

17. Signature and Title of Editor, Publisher, Business Manager, or Owner

[signature] Jody Tanach – Executive Director of Subscription Services

Date September 15, 2008

I certify that all information furnished on this form is true and complete. I understand that anyone who furnishes false or misleading information on this form or who omits material or information requested on the form may be subject to criminal sanctions (including fines and imprisonment) and/or civil sanctions (including civil penalties).

PS Form 3526, September 2006 (Page 2 of 3)

Moving?

Make sure your subscription moves with you!

To notify us of your new address, find your **Clinics Account Number** (located on your mailing label above your name), and contact customer service at:

E-mail: elspcs@elsevier.com

800-654-2452 (subscribers in the U.S. & Canada)
314-453-7041 (subscribers outside of the U.S. & Canada)

Fax number: 314-523-5170

Elsevier Periodicals Customer Service
11830 Westline Industrial Drive
St. Louis, MO 63146

*To ensure uninterrupted delivery of your subscription, please notify us at least 4 weeks in advance of move.